BMAT Past Paper
Worked Solutions

Volume Two

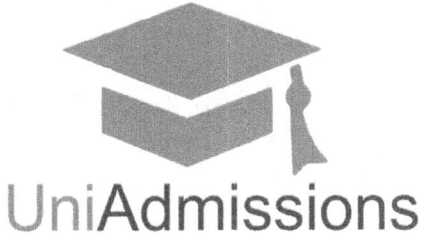

UniAdmissions

Published by *RAR Medical Services Limited*
www.uniadmissions.co.uk
info@uniadmissions.co.uk
Tel: 0208 068 0438

BMAT Past Paper
Worked Solutions

Volume Two

Somil Desai
Rohan Agarwal

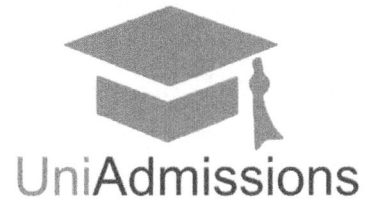

UniAdmissions

About the Authors

Somil is currently studying Accelerated Medicine at Worcester College, Oxford and hopes to one day become a Psychiatrist. Previously, Somil studied Natural Sciences at St John's College, Cambridge where he came top of the year in his final exams.

Between his 2 degrees, Somil spent a year tutoring thirty students GCSE and A Level Maths and Science, and helped several students with their Oxbridge and medical school application. Of note, he has assisted several of his tutees in exceeding their expected BMAT score.

Somil has been part of the UniAdmissions team since 2014 and has thoroughly enjoyed his work with them. In his spare time, Somil enjoys running and playing tennis.

Rohan is the **Director of Operations** at *UniAdmissions* and is responsible for its technical and commercial arms. He graduated from Gonville and Caius College, Cambridge and is a fully qualified doctor. Over the last five years, he has tutored hundreds of successful Oxbridge and Medical applicants. He has also authored ten books on admissions tests and interviews.

Rohan has taught physiology to undergraduates and interviewed medical school applicants for Cambridge. He has published research on bone physiology and writes education articles for the Independent and Huffington Post. In his spare time, Rohan enjoys playing the piano and table tennis.

THE BASICS

What are BMAT Past Papers?

Thousands of students take the BMAT exam each year. These exam papers are then released online to help future students prepare for the exam. Before 2013, these papers were not publically available meaning that students had to rely on the specimen papers and other resources for practice. However, since their release in 2013, BMAT past papers have become an invaluable resource in any student's preparation.

Where can I get BMAT Past Papers?

This book does not include BMAT past paper questions because it would be over 1,000 pages long if it did! However, all BMAT past papers since 2003 available for free from the official BMAT website. To save you the hassle of downloading lots of files, we've put them all into one easy-to-access folder for you at **www.uniadmission-s.co.uk/bmat-past-papers**.

At the time of publication, the 2017 paper has not been released so this book only contains answers for 2003 – 2016. An updated version will be made available once the 2017 paper is released. The 2014 past paper worked solutions are also available at the link above.

How should I use BMAT Past Papers?

BMAT Past papers are one the best ways to prepare for the BMAT. Careful use of them can dramatically boost your scores in a short period of time. The way you use them will depend on your learning style and how much time you have until the exam date but here are some general pointers:

➢ 4-8 weeks of preparation is usually sufficient for most students.

➢ Students generally improve in section 2 more quickly than section 1 so if you have limited time, focus on section 2.

➢ The BMAT syllabus changed in 2009 so if you find seemingly strange questions in the earlier papers, ensure you check to see if the topic is still on the specification.

➢ Similarly, there is little point doing essays before 2009 as they are significantly different in style. We've included plans for them in this book for completeness in any case.

How should I prepare for the BMAT?

Although this is a cliché, the best way to prepare for the exam is to start early – ideally by September at the latest. If you're organised and sitting the BMAT in November, you can follow the schema below:

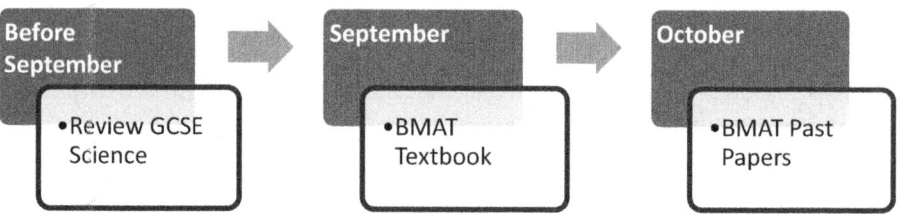

If you're sitting the BMAT in September then just move everything earlier by two months! This paradigm allows you to minimise gaps in your knowledge before you start practicing with BMAT style questions in a textbook. In general, aim to get a textbook that has lots of practice questions e.g. *The Ultimate BMAT Guide* (**www.uniadmissions.co.uk/bmat-book**) – this allows you to rapidly identify any weaknesses that you might have e.g. Newtonian mechanics, simultaneous equations etc.

You are strongly advised to get a copy of '*The Ultimate BMAT Guide*' which has 800 practice questions– you can get a free copy by following the instructions at the back of this book.

Finally, it's then time to move onto past papers. The number of BMAT papers you can do will depend on the time you have available but you should try to do at least 2009 – 2017 once.

If you have time, do 2003- 2008 once (ignore section 3). If you find that you've exhausted all past papers, there are an additional 8 mock papers available in *BMAT Practice Papers* (flick to the back to get a free copy).

How should I use this book?

This book is designed to accelerate your learning from BMAT past papers. Avoid the urge to have this book open alongside a past paper you're seeing for the first time. The BMAT is difficult because of the intense time pressure it puts you under – the best way of replicating this is by doing past papers under strict exam conditions (no half measures!). Don't start out by doing past papers (see previous page) as this 'wastes' papers.

Once you've finished, take a break and then mark your answers. Then, review the questions that you got wrong followed by ones which you found tough/spent too much time on. This is the best way to learn and with practice, you should find yourself steadily improving. You should keep a track of your scores on the next page so you can track your progress.

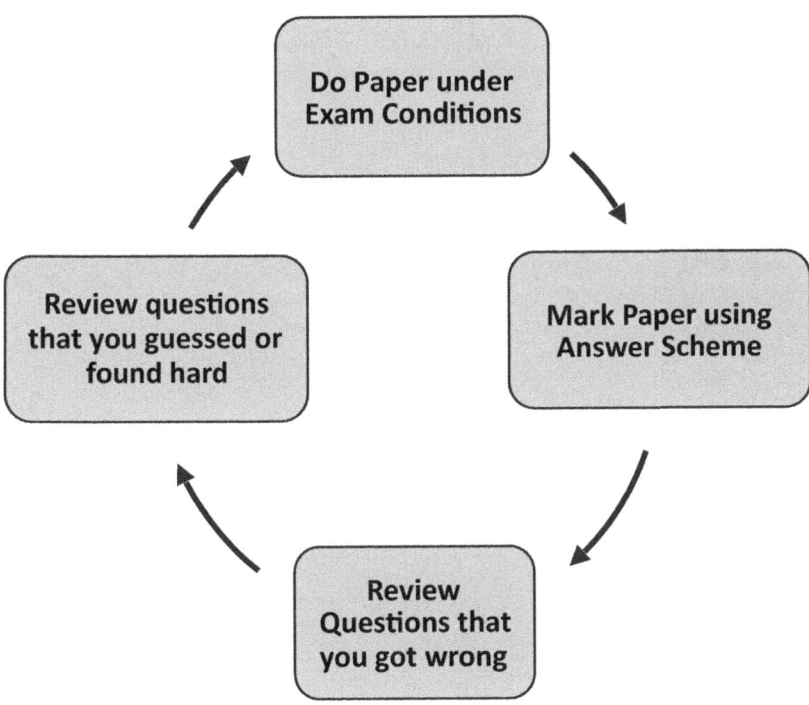

Do Paper under Exam Conditions

Mark Paper using Answer Scheme

Review Questions that you got wrong

Review questions that you guessed or found hard

Remember! You can get a free copy of Volume 1 (Papers 2003 to 2010) of BMAT *Past Paper Worked Solutions* by flicking to the back of this book.

Scoring Tables

Use these to keep a record of your scores – you can then easily see which paper you should attempt next (always the one with the lowest score).

	SECTION 1	1st Attempt	2nd Attempt	3rd Attempt
Volume One	2003			
	2004			
	2005			
	2006			
	2007			
	2008			
	2009			
	2010			
Volume Two	2011			
	2012			
	2013			
	2014			
	2015			
	2016			
	2017			

	SECTION 2	1st Attempt	2nd Attempt	3rd Attempt
	2003			
	2004			

Volume One	2005
	2006
	2007
	2008
	2009
	2010
Volume Two	2011
	2012
	2013
	2014
	2015
	2016
	2017

Extra Practice

If you're blessed with a good memory, you might remember the answers to certain questions in the past papers – making it less useful to repeat them again. If you want to tackle extra mock papers which are fully up-to-date then check out *BMAT Practice Papers* for **8** x full mock papers with worked solutions.

SECTION 1	1st Attempt	2nd Attempt	3rd Attempt
Paper A			
Paper B			
Paper C			

Paper D

Paper E

Paper F

Paper G

Paper H

SECTION 2	1st Attempt	2nd Attempt	3rd Attempt
Paper A			
Paper B			
Paper C			
Paper D			
Paper E			
Paper F			
Paper G			
Paper H			

Remember! You can get a free copy of *BMAT Practice Papers* by flicking to the back of this book.

2011

Section 1

Question 1: D

Assign each row to a bar chart based on relative values and values that are the same. Max temperature is E, wind speed is C, rain is B and cloud cover is A. D remains.

Question 2: E

None of the answers are conclusions that can be drawn from the passage.

A implies a causation between the noise of modern human life and extinction which is not a conclusion of the passage.

The passage doesn't suggest sea-based wind farms shouldn't be built so B is wrong. 'Should not' is a very bold statement and is usually involved in an incorrect answer.

Although the passage mentions that the whales are trying to adapt their communication methods, 'will be able to adapt' is too strong a phrase and thus C is wrong.

D is tempting but there is nothing to suggest that the depletion was initially caused by the growth of human noise.

Question 3: C

There is lots of irrelevant information in this question, but the maths is quite easy. Deluxe rooms are $80 a night, but there is $15 less per night being paid for no meals, so that is $65 x 6 for the room. Hiring a car is $5 + $5 x 6 (there is no taxi use). $65 x 6 + $5 + $5 x 6 = $425.

Question 4: E

The argument assumes that children either interact with each other OR play computer games, so E is correct. The other answers may be 'correct' from your previous knowledge but are unrelated to the argument. The argument is about the link between children playing computer games and social interaction, which the other answers do not address.

Question 5: F

This can be visualised to rule out 1 and 2. Also, 1 is the same as the right hand mirror, and 2 is a rotated version of the left hand mirror, which means they cannot be reflected images.

Question 6: C
The conclusion of the passage is "so all that learning…increases their memory power." This suggests that the fact their brain areas related to memory are more developed is through being a taxi driver rather than their predispositions. The other answers are not assumptions that are made in the argument.

Question 7: A
You can start by ruling out C, E and F as the range of miles per journey is too low. Out of the rest, you must work out the best fuel consumption per passenger mile. You can do this by finding out the lowest value of: fuel consumption of empty plane + fuel consumption per passenger x number of passengers. If we use 177 passengers and the values for each plane, it is easy to see that A will be the lowest per mile.

Question 8: D
Women in their 40s or 50s earned over 20% less than men on average, meaning they earned less than £0.80 for every £1 earned by a man in that range. A cannot be reliably concluded as we only have information about relative pay rather than absolute pay. B cannot be concluded, as we don't have definite information about how willing employers are to employ women based on age. C cannot be concluded, as we don't know the difference between the pay gap at the ages of 22 and 30; we only have information for the whole ranges (22-29 and 30-39).

Question 9: C
If we call male pay m, we see from the equation given that:

$$22.8 = \frac{100(m - 16000)}{m}$$

$$\frac{22.8}{100} = \frac{m - 16000}{m}$$

$$0.228m = m - 16000$$

$$0.772m = 16000$$

$$m = \frac{16000}{0.772} 20700$$

Question 10: C
The assumption is that the long hours and intensity of senior positions deterred mothers in particular, but they would be happy to take these positions in any other case, which is said in C. The other answers are irrelevant.

Question 11: D

Is the only answer that could be correct, and satisfies the maths too: using estimates we know (15-9)/15 x 100 = 40%. There is no information about part-time workers over 60 so A cannot be correct. B and C assume that absolute wage values are known, whereas we only have relative proportions.

Question 12: D

There are 6 types: fully white, fully black, ¼ outlined, ¼ outlined, ¼ black, ¼ black with the other quarters outlined.

Question 13: B

Would definitely strengthen the HAR1 hypothesis. A lack of native HAR1 causes language impairment, suggesting that it is necessary for human language ability.

A, if anything, would weaken the hypothesis as the hypothesis suggests that it is the uniqueness of HAR1 that allows human language ability.

C, D and E don't strengthen the hypothesis as they are irrelevant to human language ability.

Question 14: C

Each team played 4 matches, and we can determine how many wins, draws and losses each team had. With 2 points, Central must have drawn 2 and lost 2. With 8, Northern must have won 2 and drawn 2. Southern must have won 1, drawn 2 and lost 1 whilst Western must have drawn 1 and lost 3. The discrepancies (3 wins and 6 losses) mean that Eastern must have won 3 and drawn 1.

Question 15: B

1 is incorrect as the argument is not about who, in particular, defines the human rights, and 3 is irrelevant to the argument. 2 is correct because the passage assumes something cannot be both a constitutional right and human right; it can only be one or the other.

Question 16: D

Area is length x width, and volume is area x depth. So, all we need here volume/width to determine the highest value for depth. Don't waste time working out answers for lakes that are not an answer, and we don't need to use exact numbers. For example, Caspian Sea's depth is 78,200/394,299 which we can think of as 80,000/400,000 which is roughly 0.2 km. When we do the same for the others, Baikal clearly has the highest depth which is around 0.67 km

Question 17: C

1 isn't an assumption made: the argument doesn't require the assumption that most of the population have eaten beef infected with BSE. In fact, the main conclusion is that there will be further outbreaks in the future as those who consumed the infected beef grow older, and this is irrelevant to how many have eaten the beef.

2 is clearly incorrect, as the argument discusses that inheriting the V variant in the M-V combination can lead to developing vCJD in later life. 3 is correct as the argument assumes the combination of genes is the most important factor rather than the M variant itself.

Question 18: B

Jasper earns £240 + £5 x 22 + £20 x 6 = £470 per week, so Ruby earns £510 per week. Ruby is 35, and if we call her years worked as y, £240 + £5 x 14 + £20 x y = £510, and y = 10. This means Ruby has worked for 4 more years than Jasper.

Question 19: A

The sum of the possible outcomes for drilling is -720000 x 0.1 + 400000 x 0.8 + 3800000 x 0.1 = $628000
The sum of possible outcomes for not drilling is 1000000 x 0.2 + 500000 x 0.6 = 500000. So drilling represents a more favourable option than not drilling.

Question 20: D

Is correct – the probability of a 'medium' strike is 0.8, as is the probability of selling the drilling rights at $500,000 or $1,000,000 (0.6 + 0.2). A is incorrect, as a medium strike allows a profit too. B is incorrect, as $400,000 x 0.8 is less than $500,000. C is incorrect, as there is only a 0.1 chance of making a loss, and a 0.9 chance (medium or big strike) of making a profit.

Question 21: F

All of the answers are correct. The costs would be £1,300,000 for drilling, which is higher than the returns for a medium strike (£1,200,000). The only way to make a profit is thus a big strike, which has a 10% chance. They could however make a profit if they reduced drilling costs by 25% to £600,000, so costs would be £1,100,000, which is lower than the returns for a medium strike.

Question 22: E

The sum of expected outcomes for drilling is $628,000 and is $500,000 for not drilling. Paying the insurance would make the value for drilling $428,000. Without insurance, the expected outcome for an oil spill is -$10,000,000 x 0.03 = $300,000, making the value for drilling $328,000. Not drilling has a value of $500,000. So, the order is 3, 1, 2.

Question 23: D

Determine which numbers haven't been used. On the left side the remaining numbers must add up to 13, and must be 6 and 7, but we don't know which order. On the right hand side they must add up to 10, so they are 8 and 2 but we don't know which order. This mean the number right of 9 must be 4, and the remaining 2 numbers must add up to 8 on this row, which must be 6 and 2. So between 5 and 3 is 7.

Question 24: A
The quote means Fredericks will not play if Petermass is fit, and may or may not play if Petermass is not fit. This makes 1 correct and 2 and 3 incorrect.

Question 25: C
The one with equal proportions has 90ml of oil and vinegar and the other has 120ml oil and 60ml vinegar. So if we add half of the one with equal proportions to the other, we have 45ml of each in the first and we have 165ml oil and 105ml vinegar in the other. This latter one represents 11/18 oil and 7/18 vinegar. If 90ml of this mix is taken, 55ml will be oil and 35ml will be vinegar. So there will be 110ml oil in one (165-55) and 100ml (45+55) in the other.

Question 26: C
This is the correct answer as the argument talks of the possibility that many planets could support human life.
➢ A is not correct as gravity is not the only factor that determines whether a planet can support life.
➢ B is not necessarily correct and the use of the word 'must' means it is probably too bold a statement.
➢ D is tempting but the passage uses the words 'probably in the order of 10 or 20 per cent', so saying it is 10 or 20 percent is too strong.
➢ E is again too bold a statement, as the passage only says that there 'could be' tens of billions of these systems.

Question 27: A
This is easier than it looks. The question is asking if you can form a 6 x 2 or a 4 x 3 rectangle with 3 of the shapes. However, it's not actually possible to form a rectangle of those dimensions regardless of the shapes you pick.

Question 28: C
2 is not necessary information for the argument; the distance that each bus needs to travel every week is irrelevant, so C must be the correct answer. We can check and see that the other points are reasonable, which they are.
Question 29: D
3km from the library is the distance when Claire leaves 20 minutes late. This tells you that when Claire leaves on time she is 1km from the library when Charles is 3km away (she walks 2km in 20 minutes so had she left on time she would be 2km further along).

As they usually meet at the Library, Charles has to cover 3km while she covers 1km, so he cycles 3 times faster than she walks at 18km/hr.

Question 30: B
Paraphrases the last 2 sentences of the passage and is the correct answer. A and D are both too bold to be answers as the passage highlights that it is just a theory. C isn't correct as we don't know if it is the best explanation – we haven't heard any other hypotheses.

Question 31: C
There are 20 cans remaining. The view from X shows us that there are 6 cans in the shaded columns remaining. Thus, there are 14 cans in the 6 columns in the middle. Thus, a maximum of 4 cans can be missing from the middle 6 columns.

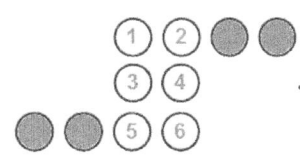

Options A, B, E and F are too full to not be possible. D is still possible if columns 3 and 4 only have one can each (therefore columns 1-6 = 14). Only C is therefore not possible as columns 1 and 2 would have to be 2 cans tall and columns 3 and 4 to be 1 can tall (6 cans missing).

Question 32: C
Rounding is ok here because of the big difference between answers. 1500 patients per doctor, so a total of 1500 x 5 consultations a year = 7500 consultations a year per doctor. 7500/250 = 30 consultations a day, and C is the closest (it would be closer to 32 if we didn't round down earlier).

Question 33: D
The proportion in 1995 was 0.8/3.29 which is close to 0.2, and was 1.8/5.26 in 2006 which is close to 0.33. The percentage increase is (0.33-0.20)/0.20 x 100 which is roughly 65%, making D the closest.

Question 34: C
C is clearly the only viable answer, as the ratio is definitely above 2 between 15 and 35 and then starts to decrease towards 1.

Question 35: C
People may have become 11 years older, but there is still the same age group within the age demographics, so ageing is irrelevant. The others are relevant.

END OF SECTION

Section 2

Question 1: F

Carbohydrase is an enzyme – not a gland, hormone or a function so does not fit into the table. All the other words/statements fit in somewhere.

Question 2: B

X has 3 electrons in its outer most electron shell and Y needs 2 electrons to make a complete outer electron shell. I.e. Valency of X is +3 and Y is -2. The easy way to figure out formulae is to 'swap' the valencies to give: X_2Y_3.

Question 3: C

Remember that $E_k = \dfrac{mv^2}{2}$ and $E_p = mg\,\Delta h$

Since E_k is proportional to velocity^2, doubling the velocity means E_k is 4 times higher. E_p is proportional to height so doubling the height means E_p is 2 times greater. Thus, C is the correct answer.

Question 4: C

$$3x\left(3x^{-\frac{1}{3}}\right)^3$$

$$= 3x\left(3^3 x^{-\frac{3}{3}}\right)$$

$$= 3x\left(27x^{-1}\right)$$

$$= 3x\left(\frac{27}{x}\right)$$

$$= 81$$

Question 5: F

Mitosis produces genetically identical cells and meiosis results in variation so 1 and 2 are wrong. Statements 3,4 and 5 are correct.

Question 6: D

Raising the temperature increases the average kinetic energy of all molecules. Thus, more collisions take place per unit time and the average collision has more energy. However, temperature has no effect on the orientation of the molecules.

Question 7: E
A. Nuclear fission is the splitting of a nucleus into 2 small parts. Whilst gamma radiation may be released, this is not the definition of fission.
B. The half life of a radioactive substance is the time taken for half of it to decay (not half the time for it to decay).
C. The number of neutrons is given by the mass number – atomic number, not the other way around.
D. Nuclear power stations utilise fission, not fusion.
E. A beta particle consists of a highly charged electron. There is no change in the atomic mass.
F. When a nucleus emits an alpha particle, it loses 2 neutrons + 2 protons.

Question 8: D
At 9:45 the hour hand will be ¾ of the way to 10 from 9 and the minutes hand will be at 9. The number of degrees between the hours is $\dfrac{360}{12} = 30$. Thus ¾ of this is 22.5 degrees.

Question 9: C
4 is incorrect because individuals with relatively disadvantageous adaptations will still usually be able to breed, unless that adaptation actually causes death or an inability to breed. The other statements are correct.

Question 10: D
Each carbon atom can make 4 bonds and each hydrogen atom can make 1 bond. So the outer carbons are bonded to 2 hydrogens each. However, the carbon atoms between the two rings are only bound to 1 hydrogen. So if we count up, there are 10 carbons and 18 hydrogens.
Thus, $A_r = (12 x 10) + (1 x 18) = 138$

Question 11: B
Be careful! The current in this circuit flows clockwise (most circuits are anticlockwise). The diode is thus a break in the circuit in this direction. When the switch is open, we have 2 breaks in the circuit, so no current can flow through either of the branches. Thus, the reading on the ammeter will be 0. When the switch is closed, the current can pass through the branch without the diode in it. Since the resistance is 3 ohms and voltage is 6V: $I = \dfrac{6}{3} = 2A$

Question 12: D

The quickest way to solve this is via trial and error- assign values to each option to see if you can disprove them e.g. If W is 3 and x is 2, then option A would be incorrect (yet the inequalities in the question would still hold). The only inequality that **must** be true is x > y because $y^2 < x$.

Question 13: E

Oxygen and carbon dioxide move across membranes via diffusion, not osmosis. Oxygenated blood goes to muscles and deoxygenated blood returns from muscles. The oxygen concentration is low in the muscle cells as oxygen is required for aerobic respiration, and carbon dioxide is high because it is produced during aerobic respiration. Thus:

➢ CO_2 is high in muscles and low in plasma.
➢ O_2 is high in RBC and low in muscle.
➢ Hence, E is correct.

Question 14: C

A metal cannot form covalent bonds with a non-metal, so NaCl and Na_2O are ionic compounds. All the other compounds contain a covalent bond.

Question 15: B

This is a good example of why it's handy to know the suvat equations as it can save you a lot of time.

Using $v^2 = u^2 + 2as$

$0^2 = 300^2 + 2xax0.6$

Thus, $0 = 90000 + 1.2a$

$a = \dfrac{9x10^4}{1.2} = 7.5x10^4$

Now use $F = ma$ to give: $F = 0.05x7.5x10^4$

$F = 0.375x10^4 = 3.75x10^3 N$

Question 16: E
Don't try to solve these algebraically – it's much quicker to sketch them!

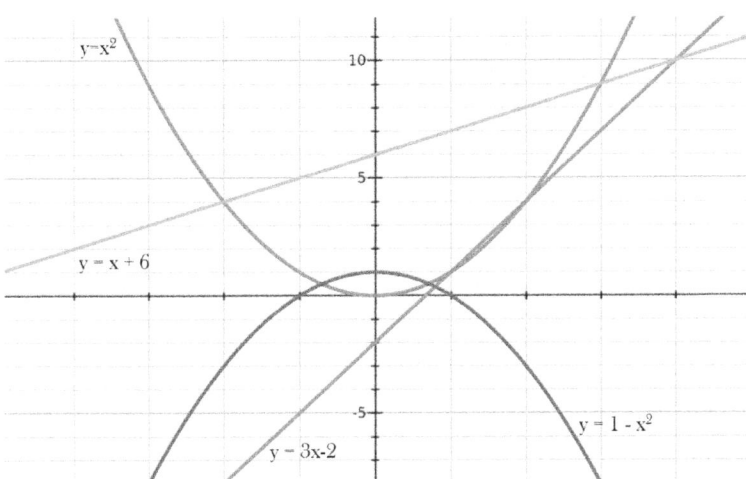

As is easily visible, $y = 1 - x^2$ and $y = x + 6$ don't intersect. Thus, the answer is E.

Question 17: D
Any are feasible. The condition could be dominant with P, Q, R and S having the recessive alleles only. The sperm from T could have carried the allele from the condition, or a mutation could have been present in an egg of S.

Question 18: E
The easiest way to solve this is to set up your own algebraic equation for Oxygen (as it appears the most number of times):
$3B = 6X + Y + 2$
Then simply see if any of the options satisfy this equation- only option E does. If you're unsure about how to setup these equations then check out the chemistry chapter in *The Ultimate BMAT Guide*.

Question 19: A
The current flowing through a resistor at a constant temperature is directly proportional to the potential difference across it. Thus, as voltage increases, current increases at a constant rate i.e. resistance does not change.

Question 20: B
This is a test of how quickly you can use Pythagoras's theorem:

Bottom Triangle:
The hypotenuse is given by $= \sqrt{1^2 + 3^2} = \sqrt{10}$
Middle Triangle:

Since the triangles are similar, the small edge must be 1/3 of $\sqrt{10} = \dfrac{\sqrt{10}}{3}$

The hypotenuse is given by $= \sqrt{\left(\sqrt{10}\right)^2 + \left(\dfrac{\sqrt{10}}{3}\right)^2} = \sqrt{10 + \dfrac{10}{9}}$

$= \sqrt{\dfrac{90 + 10}{9}} = \sqrt{\dfrac{100}{9}} = \dfrac{10}{3}$

Top Triangle:
Since the triangles are similar, the small edge must be 1/3 of $\dfrac{10}{3} = \dfrac{10}{9}$

The area of the triangle $= \frac{1}{2} base x height = \dfrac{1}{2} x \dfrac{10}{9} x \dfrac{10}{3}$

$= \dfrac{100}{54} = \dfrac{50}{27} cm^2$

Question 21: D
Cell P is haploid and can be any sex cell. Cell Q is diploid and can be almost any somatic cell. Cell R can be enucleated, or a red blood cells (because they have no nucleus). Only D satisfies these criteria.

Question 22: D
The mass of PbS in the ore $= 70\% of 478kg$
$= \dfrac{70}{100} x 478 = 335kg$
The atomic mass of PbS $= 207 + 32 = 239$
The proportion of lead in PbS $= \dfrac{207}{239} \approx \dfrac{210}{240} = 0.875$
Thus, the mass of lead that can be extracted $= 0.875 x 335 = 293kg$
The closest answer to this is 289.8 kg.

NB: Remember rounding numbers to make the maths easier also means you won't get the **exact** answer on the paper. Thus, always check the options to see how much room you have to round numbers. If they are close together then you should avoid rounding and vice versa.

Question 23: C

Light travels slower in glass than air, but its frequency remains the same. Since $c = f$, wavelength must decrease to accommodate for the lower speed. Option C is the only one that satisfies these requirements.

Question 24: B

12 can only be achieved by rolling 2 sixes.

The probability of rolling a 6 on the fair die = 1/6

$$P(12) = P(6 on fair die) x P(6 on unfair die)$$

$$\frac{1}{18} = \frac{1}{6} x P(6 on unfair die)$$

Thus, $P(6 on unfair die) = \frac{1}{3}$

$$P\left(1 to 5 on unfair die\right) = 1 - \frac{1}{3} = \frac{2}{3}$$

$$P\left(1 on unfair die\right) = \frac{\frac{2}{3}}{5} = \frac{2}{15}$$

2 can only be achieved by rolling 2 ones.

$$P(2) = P\left(1 on fair die\right) x P\left(1 on unfair die\right) = \frac{2}{15} x \frac{1}{6}$$

Simplifies to: $\frac{1}{90} = \frac{1}{45}$

Question 25: D

The homeostatic response brings the level back to the stable, normal level. If the system is less responsive, all phases are likely to occur later (not earlier) and the deviation from the normal level will be higher.   Thus, phase 2 would be higher.

Question 26: E

The key word here is **excess** oxygen. When sulphur reacts with oxygen, the product is Sulphur dioxide. This eliminates options A-C.

Since there is excess oxygen, the other product will be carbon dioxide (not carbon monoxide). Thus, E is correct.

Question 27: B

50 beats per minute means there is a beat every $\frac{6}{5}$ seconds. Since the back soldiers put down their left foot at the same time as the front soldiers put down their right, the adjusted beat is every $\frac{3}{5}$ seconds.

Thus, the $minimum\ distance = \dfrac{3}{5} x\,330 = \dfrac{990}{5} = 198$ m

END OF SECTION

SECTION THREE

Section 3

"Democratic freedom means there should be no restriction on what may be said in public."

> Democracy allows power to be vested in the people; it perpetuates the idea of freedom, equality and liberty, and thus the right of expression including freedom of speech. This suggests there should be no restriction or intervention if someone wishes to express their opinion in a public setting.

> Freedom of speech does not necessarily remove all boundaries; a restriction on the proclamation of unwarranted, extreme and prejudiced ideas seems just.

> People generally believe what they hear from people that appear more 'powerful' than them. Giving misleading information to the public can be dangerous; for example, the freedom to preach that drink-driving is not a crime to a bar could endanger many.

> Complete freedom of speech allows those with extreme ideas to declare whatever they believe, which could be to the detriment of young, impressionable minds enticed by these opinions.

> There should be a limit if 'free speech' is inciting hatred. Discrimination against minorities, whether it is sexuality, race or even age, can cause friction, hatred and 'broken' societies that is against the very notion of a democratic society.

> A utilitarian stance appears fairest; the 'harm principle' postulates that the actions of individuals should only be limited to those that prevent harm to other individuals, and this appears a good balance between completely free speech and a restrictive stranglehold. A difference in opinion can and should be freely expressed, but it is explicable that hate speech, classified information, obscenity, etc. is regulated.

The art of medicine consists of amusing the patient while nature cures the disease.

➢ The author argues the point that medicine is an art, and suggests that physicians need qualities of empathy and compassion to help satisfy patients' worries and beliefs while nature takes its course to cure them over time.

➢ Although this statement may have been wholly true in the 18th century, nowadays medicine is an applied science and it is debatable whether the statement still has any implications for the doctors of today.

➢ Scientific knowledge now allows us to treat patients better or more quickly than nature. Drugs target specific biochemical or physiological systems in order to cure. The fact that clinical trials are double blind and tested against a placebo and require a statistically significant difference between the groups highlights that the active ingredient of a drug is having an effect greater than that of nature and the 'amusing' of a patient. Example of the swine flu pandemic in 2009; oseltamivir highly successful. Many infectious diseases through history are now effectively eradicated worldwide.

➢ However, placebo is much more effective than no treatment, suggesting that patients can seek comfort in the thought that they are being cared for by those who they believe have the knowledge and skill to do so.

➢ Example of the common cold – can only treat the symptoms and wait for the innate immune system to take control.

➢ Doctors must always use more than science; examples include the importance of teamwork, leadership and diagnosis where there is no scientific method except interacting with the patient (e.g. bipolar disorder and other psychiatric illnesses).

A scientific man ought to have no wishes, no affections - a mere heart of stone.

➢ Darwin tackles the issue of objectivity in science; the ability to remain unbiased and develop conclusions true to our empirical evidence rather than true to our beliefs. Wishes and affections greatly influence one's behaviour and one's rationality.

➢ Within science there undoubtedly exists a facet which requires absolute removal of our wishes and affections. These traits could influence experiments and therefore could and render invalid the interpretations of these studies, which would be detrimental in our aim to dispel our own ignorance and further scientific knowledge. There are many examples of where passion and bias have blinded scientists to that which has been objectively proven. A famous example is Sir Fred Hoyle who rejected Hawking's presentation of the Big Bang Theory despite overwhelming evidence (cosmic microwave background) until his death.

➢ It can be dangerous to not show complete objectivity. An example is the case of Andrew Wakefield, the gentlemen who asserted the link between the MMR vaccine and the onset of autism, which resulted in the deaths of many children from measles, mumps and rubella. (AW falsified his results and subjected autistic subjects to unethical procedures to 'prove' that the MMR vaccine causes autism after being bribed by a law firm that was planning on suing the MMR vaccine company. After repeat experiments were performed and the results acquired were found to be completely different, AW's paper was withdrawn from the Lancet and he was struck off the medical register.) Sadly, the myth that MMR vaccines cause autism is still believed and herd immunity has not reached pre-scare levels. Scientists should thus welcome other scientists with different prejudices and preferences to follow what they have done to see if they get the same results through peer reviewing.

➢ But our objectivity is not intended to quash our biases and natural passion and yearning for a scientific outcome. On the contrary, objectivity very much allows us to be passionate for science because it prevents the passion from influencing the results. So why have passion at all? Passion, drive and intrigue are intrinsic to scientific discovery and enquiry. Without such qualities Fleming or Darwin might never have discovered antibiotics and evolution. Einstein has always asserted the importance of imagination over knowledge. One reason is that imagination and creativity allows for options for technological advances that were unplanned and unprecedented (e.g. Fleming).

➢ One could argue that this is oxymoronic, as if one is "a scientific man" this suggests they have an affection and wish to proceed with scientific method. Without our wishes and affections, there would be no driving force underpinning our desire to understand how the world works.

Veterinary pet care in the UK should be free at the point of delivery, as human care is.

> The argument is that, as sentient beings, animals should receive free healthcare like their human owners.

> Animals experience disease, pain and illness in the (arguably) same manner that we do, and our experience with these should mean our empathy extends to the animal world. The mantra of public healthcare is essentially that everyone deserves the 'right' of healthcare, regardless of wealth, status and privilege. Should this not translate to animals that are often most vulnerable?

> For most owners, their pet is part of the family and they would do anything to protect them and ensure they stay healthy.

> This plan would reduce the number if abandoned pets whose owners were unable to afford veterinary care.

> One of the core responsibilities of pet ownership is that you should make sure that you can take care of them and can afford to pay for everything that they need for the entire duration of their lives. If one cannot afford veterinary care, then perhaps they should not have a pet. In any case, taking out pet insurance is recommended to most owners.

> Public healthcare through the NHS is only possible in the UK because taxpayers contribute towards its funding. In the case of veterinary care, forcing non-pet owners to pay taxes towards other people's pets - essentially, for a service that they will not use - seems very unfair. However, we do pay for the healthcare of those who smoke, heavily drink or take part in extreme sports, which is similarly 'unfair' in the sense that they are much more likely to use the publically funded money than others. Owners may agree to pay a kind of specific owner tax.

> It is also possible that pet owners may take less responsibility for their pet's health if they know that they will not have to pay for veterinary care.

> It is hard to draw a line between how well we should treat animals relative to ourselves. It is clear that in general we treat ourselves as if we are 'above' animals in society; we eat them, we test on them and we exploit them. If we have the re-

sources to keep them healthy, then they deserve to have free healthcare, but this may be at the expense of other resources that the majority of people find more important in a democratic society.

END OF PAPER

SECTION ONE

2012

Section 1

Question 1: D

10% of the population is 8628709 x 0.1 = 862870.9, and the only islands with less than this amount are Brosnan and Dalton. 20% of the area is 26315 x 0.2 = 5263; Brosnan has less than this amount and Dalton has more, so the answer is Dalton.

HINT: As only 1 answer can be correct, for the second part of this question it can be assumed that the higher value is above 20% and the lower value is below 20% without doing any exact workings.

Question 2: C

As it is preceded by the words '*based on these findings*,' it is fairly easy to determine that the main conclusion of the passage is "*pale-skinned people should be added to the list of those for whom vitamin D supplements are recommended by the government.*"

- ➣ A could probably be argued as correct based on the passage with a lack of a better answer, but the conclusion above clearly mentions supplements which this answer does not. Furthermore, the use of the word 'need' immediately suggests that the answer is probably too strong and thus incorrect.
- ➣ B is probably true based on the information, but again is a point made to back up the argument rather than the main conclusion of the passage.
- ➣ C paraphrases the conclusion given above, and is clearly the best answer.
- ➣ D may be tempting from your previous knowledge, but is irrelevant and beyond the scope of this passage as skin cancer is not mentioned.
- ➣ E is not correct as the passage makes no comparison between pale and dark skinned people. Again, we can probably rule this answer out from the start for being too strong and sweeping.

Question 3: F

The best way to answer this question is probably by testing the effect of eliminating each tile. Checking whether the number of black and white tiles is equal first is probably easiest as they stand out, but if this criterion is satisfied the other patterns must be checked too.

➤ By removing A, you can see that you will be left with 6 black tiles and only 4 white tiles.

➤ Removing B leaves 5 black tiles but 6 white tiles.

➤ Removing C leaves 3 black tiles but 5 white tiles.

➤ Removing D leaves 6 black tiles and only 5 white tiles.

➤ Removing E leaves 5 black tiles and 5 white tiles. However, only 3 of the dotted pattern remain.

Removing F leaves 5 black tiles and 5 white tiles. It can also be seen that all the other patterns amount to 5 tiles.

Question 4: B

This question asks for a conclusion of the passage.

A can be inferred but is not a conclusion of the passage.

B is the best answer as it sums up one of the fundamental points of the argument, "*only fossil fuels, which produce emissions of CO_2, can provide the extra capacity.*"

The use of the word 'never' in C immediately suggests that this is the incorrect answer, and there is no mention of the future potential of wind power.

D is incorrect, as the first sentence states that electric engines are actually more economical than petrol engines.

Question 5: E

The best way to answer this question is to work out the collective area of the shrubs, veg, pond and lawn, take this away from the total area and then determine the number of slabs needed. We are given several widths and heights of these areas and must work out the other ones.

➤ The height of the pond is equal to the veg (3m) and is clearly a square, so the area of the pond is $3 \times 3 = 9m^2$

➤ The total width of the veg areas is $18 - 1 - 3 - 1 - 0.5 - 0.5 - 1 = 11$, therefore the total area of these plots are $11 \times 3 = 33m^2$

➤ The total width that the shrubs take up is $18 - 1 - 3 - 1 - 0.5 - 1 = 11.5m$, thus the total area that the shrubs take up is $4 \times 11.5 = 46m^2$

➤ The height that the lawn takes up is $12 - 1 - 3 - 1 - 1 = 6m$, so the area of the lawn is $3 \times 6 = 18cm^2$

➤ The total area of the garden is $18 \times 12 = 216m^2$, so the area taken up by the patio and paths is $216 - 9 - 33 - 46 - 18 = 110m^2$

➤ $1m^2$ requires 4 ($0.5m^2$) slabs, so $110m^2$ requires $110 \times 4 = 440$ slabs.

Question 6: E

The main conclusion of the argument is *"if parents spend time discussing these issues with their children they will help their children read well,"* given away by the use of the word 'so' and the fact that it is at the end of the passage. (As a general rule, conclusions are more likely to be at the start or end of a passage than in the middle). Flaws are generally related to the conclusion of the passage, whereas questions asking for statements that 'weaken' the argument could potentially relate to any of the passage.

➤ A is clearly wrong as there is no mention of peer groups in the passage, and the statement has nothing to do with the conclusion above.

➤ B could be maybe be debated, but appears like a weak suggestion in the face of other flaws given, and is not directly related to the conclusion of the argument.

➤ C again could maybe be argued, but is again not linked to the conclusion of the argument, and there is clearly a more pertinent answer.

➤ D is unrelated to the conclusion and is beyond the scope of the passage.

➤ E is the best answer, as it directly addresses the conclusion above. A key principle in scientific argument, and hence the BMAT, is that correlation $\neq$ causation, which this statement asserts.

Question 7: A

This is a very difficult question, and you should ensure that you do not spend over 2 minutes trying to work this out and drawing all the permutations. For pattern questions like this it is best to work out what you must add to carry on repeating the pattern indefinitely (the 'repeating unit'. This repeating unit consists of 1 hexagon, 2 triangles and 3 squares.

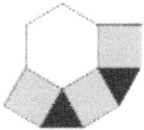

The easy way to do this was to realise that there are more squares than triangles in the diagram- this allows you to eliminate B,C and D. Intuitively, it is unlikely to be E (as that is obtained just by counting all the shapes)- leaving you with A as the only option.

Question 8: C

In questions like this it is too time-consuming to work with exact numbers and the best method is to work with close estimates. The total number of patient days we are dealing with is 11549 + 30432 = around 42000.

Method 1: The rate of infection is 9.86 per 10000 over ~30000 patient days, so over ~40000 days it will be ¾ of this value, which is slightly under 7.5, and 7.15 appears a very reasonable answer.

Method 2: There are 3 cases in 42000 days. To make this per 100000 days we have to times the number of cases by roughly. This equals 7.5 and again 7.15 appears the correct solution.

Question 9: D

The highest number of cases by far comes from organisation 3, with 26. This is out of a total of 69 (you can probably work this out using mental maths to save time). 26/69 is not intuitive, so we can use short division to work out that the first 3 digits are 0.37, suggesting that 38% is the correct answer of the ones listed.

HINT: We know that 69/3 is 23, thus 23/69 is equivalent to 1/3 or 33%. Our answer is higher than this value so we can easily rule out answers A-C.

Question 10: B
Again, don't waste time by working out exact values and use rough estimates.
- Organisation 2 had $16000/11 = \sim 1500$ patient days per month up to November, giving a total of 17500 for the year.
- We thus have 1 case in 17500 days but we need a value per 100000 days.
- $100000/17500 = 100/17.5$.
- $100/17.5$ is clearly between 5 and 6 as we know $100/5 = 20$ and $100/6 = 16.7$. This is an easy way of ruling out C-E.
- We must then determine whether A or B is correct. We can work out that $17.5 \times 5 = 87.5$ and $17.5 \times 6 = 105$. 100 is closer to the latter, which means the answer is above 5.5 and thus must be 5.67.

Question 11: E
- E is the correct answer, which we can determine by ruling out all of the other statements.

  A & C - Several of the organisations are made up of more than 1 type of hospital, and the data is not split between these so we don't know which type of hospital the cases were found in. We can thus not reliably conclude where these Cdl cases occurred.
- B - There is only 1 organisation with a small hospital alone, and this had only 1 case over 2009 and 2010 with a low rate of infection, so this is definitely incorrect.
- D - Again, using the reasoning above, there may not necessarily have been any Cdl found in either DCs or TCs. For example, only organisation 5 has a DC in the data given and here, all the cases may have arisen from the TC.

Question 12: B
Nicola wants to get the first bus of the day from the airport, which is at 09:15 on Thursday. It takes 50 minutes to get to the centre, so she will be there at 10:05. She must get the 15:20 bus from the centre to reach the airport before 17:00. Thus she is in the centre between 10:05 to 15:20, which is 15:20 - 10:05 = 5 hours and 15 minutes.

Question 13: D

This question should hopefully be relatively easy based on the BMAT tricks and tips you have learnt thus far. The correct letter can be determined just from reading the answers, as the passage is relatively passive and unforceful in its conclusions, whereas 3 of the answers are far too strong.

> A uses the word 'only' and C uses the word 'must' which suggests they are wrong, and the passage is much less bold than these statements.

> B is slightly less strong but the use of 'would not have' means the answer is not necessarily true, especially with a better answer present.

> D is not overly strong and paraphrases the first sentence, making it the best answer.

Question 14: D

The cube must be visualised to work out this question. A and B can be ruled out because the triangle should always point to the long end of a solid line. C and E are excluded by looking at the configuration of the X and the surrounding shapes. If you get stuck and have time, make the net yourself – it will save time in the long run.

Question 15: C

The conclusion of this argument is "*parents of children with autism are damaging their children's health by using the sprays*," and the rest is background information.

> A would actually support this conclusion and does not weaken the argument

> B would again strengthen the argument as it reinforces the idea that parents are potentially damaging children if preliminary tests have not been done.

> C is the best answer, as if it were true, the claim in the conclusion becomes much less convincing.

> D isn't directly relevant to the question and doesn't potentially weaken the argument depending on what these cultural effects entail and is therefore not the right answer.

> E also strengthens the argument by suggesting that oxytocin is bad.

Question 16: C

To make this question easier, we can focus on 1/6th of the conservatory as it represents the pattern of the whole area. There are 25 tiles in this area, of which 5 have the pattern with no black, 4 have the pattern with ¼ black, 12 have the pattern which is ½ black and 4 have the pattern with all black.

To work out the proportion of black, we need to work out the number of black tiles that these tiles add up to, and divide it by the total number of tiles. 0 x 5 + 0.25 x 4 + 0.5 x 12 + 1 x 4 = 11, and dividing this by 25 (times by 4 and divide by 100) is 0.44 (44%).

Question 17: G

None of the statements can be drawn as a conclusion of the passage.

1 - This is a strong statement and although the passage states staffing levels are lower

at weekends and there are more deaths at weekends, it does not suggest the causation that increased staffing would reduce death rates.

2 – The passage states that patients are dying in hospitals rather than at home (which implies that they would die anyway). This artificially inflates the mortality stats. Thus, enhancing weekend provision of primary care services wouldn't help mortality rates-only massage the statistics.

3 - This again assumes the causation that low staffing levels leads to patient deaths, which is not what the passage suggests.

Question 18: A

If x is the percentage of people that own both a tumble dryer and a dishwasher, we must work out the smallest and largest possible values of x.

75 to 85 - x is the number of people with only a dishwasher, 35to40 - x is the number of people with only a tumble dryer, 0to5 is the number of people with neither and x is the number of people with both. Thus 75to85 - x + 35to40 - x + x + 0to5 = 100, meaning x = 75to85 + 35to40 + 0to5 - 100.

Smallest value: x = 75 + 35 + 0 - 100 = 10%, largest value: x = 85 + 40 + 5 = 30%

Question 19: B

The number of category A calls in 2011 was 2.23 million. 74.9% (we can take this as 75%) were responded to within 8 minutes, leaving 25% not responded to within 8 minutes. 2.23 x 0.25 is slightly above 0.5, and working it out fully gives an answer of 0.5575.

Question 20: D

We are told that category A calls made up around 34%, category B calls made up roughly 40% and so category C calls made up the remainder (26%). We thus want a pie chart showing Category C taking up very slightly more than a quarter of the graph and category A taking up around a third. Only pie chart D fits this bill.

Question 21: B

➢ **B is** the only sensible answer.

➢ A is completely irrelevant to how many calls led to treatment/transport at the scene.

➢ C suggests that something being a 'genuine emergency' completely determines whether people are treated/transported at a scene, which is not the case. B is the better answer.

➢ D is wrong as category C cases may still require treatment/transport, but with different timings. Also, 26% of calls were category C, which amounts to over 2 million.

Question 22: A

In 2010, 2.08 million incidents were category A, and ~75% were attended within 8 minutes. 2.08 x 0.75 = 1.56m

In 2011, 2.23 million incidents were category B, and ~75% were attended within 8 minutes. 2.23 x 0.75 = 1.68m

1.68 - 1.56 = 0.12 million

Question 23: B

Working horizontally, we can see that patterns 1, 3, 8 and 10 are equivalent, patterns 6, 7 and 11 are equivalent and patterns 4 and 12 are equivalent. This leaves patterns 2, 5 and 9. 2 and 9 are equivalent through rotation, but pattern 5 cannot be rotated to match either of these. There are thus 5 distinct patterns.

Question 24: E

The conclusion is clearly the first line: "*Police should be given clear permission to use water cannons against rioters and rules about when it is appropriate.*"

➢ A weakens the argument as it suggests that water cannons also affecting the innocent means it is not a good solution for targeting crime.

➢ B could maybe be debated as the answer, but the police are unlikely to be against the use of training and resources.

➢ C weakens the arguments as it suggests there are other equally useful strategies.

➢ D mentions the high expense of water cannons and thus weakens the argument.

➢ E is the best answer based on the information given, as it strengthens the idea that water cannons should be used.

Question 25: C

We can work out that the highest score in a full turn is 18 and the lowest is 2, which gives 17 possible scores. We must then work out if any scores between 2 and 18 are not possible (and we only need one example of a score being possible).

2 - 2, 2, miss.

3 - 2, miss, 2

4 - 4, 4, miss
5 - 4, 6, miss

The rest of the even numbers can be made with combinations of 2, 4 and 6

7 - 6, miss, 4

9 - 6, miss, 6
Higher odd numbers cannot be made, leaving 13 possibilities in total.

Question 26: D

This argument makes the reasoning error of x is z, y is z so z is x. There may be cases of z that are not x, or z may not link to x at all.
> A follows x is y and y is z so x is z, which is reasonable.
> B suggests x is y and z so everything z is y, which is wrong but a different error to that in the passage
> C suggests x is y so not-x is not-y, which is (generally) fairly reasonable and definitely different to the reasoning error in the argument.
> D follows x is z and y is z so x is z, which is the same reasoning argument as above.

Question 27: C

We know that furniture costs 3 months to pay, with ½ paid in the 1st month, and ¼ in the next 2 - this means that it does not matter whether sales of e.g. $2000 came from 1 sale or from several sales, as the money received per month will be equivalent in either case. We also know that there were no sales in May and June. Using these 2 pieces of information we can deduce the answer.

June must have been the final payment for 1 piece/pieces of furniture due to the closure, which means $2000 must also have come in from this April sale in May and $4000 in April. This gives a total of $8000 of sales from April

The extra $1000 in April and May earned must have come from a sale in March, which would have amounted to a total of $4000 in March, and a total of $2000 earned from this/these sales in March.

The $2000 missing from March must have come from January sales of $8000, giving $4000 in January and $2000 in February. Any excess money from January and February must have come from furniture sold before January.

Thus, the total sales in this time period are $8000 (January), $4000 (March) and $8000 (April), giving an answer of $20000.

Question 28: G

All the answers identify a weakness in the argument.

1. This is a weakness as saying "*this is nonsense*" suggests that the author thinks the ski holiday industry does not damage the environment, because all travel damages the environment.
2. This is a weakness as the argument that ski holiday resorts use less energy than other resorts is conflicted by this information. Using percentages here may mask the fact that absolute levels of energy consumption may be high, which this statement addresses
3. This is definitely a weakness as the author fails to consider that damage to the environment is not only caused by energy consumption.

Question 29: C

➢ £12240 was made from y sales.
➢ 0.4y represents 40% of the ticket sales that were refunded £5 each.
➢ So 0.6y x 20 + 0.4y x 15 = 12240. Solving for x gives x=680.
➢ 40% of 680 is 272 tickets, and £5 x 272 = £1360 refunded.

Question 30: C

Only statement 3 can be inferred. This could maybe be determined without the passage as it is least bold statement.

1 - "*authors...give a one sided view*" is very strong and the passage does not mention effectiveness or safety.

2 - There is nothing to suggest that "*companies...aim to influence the content of the articles.*"

3 - This effectively paraphrases what is said in the first 2 sentences of the passage.

Question 31: C

We can deduce several things from this passage:

We know Jill must be at least 7 points ahead of 4th place so that even if she comes last and they come first the places remain the same. With the same reasoning, she must also be at least 7 points behind 2nd place.

Karen and Gemma must have the same number of points, so that even if one comes 3rd and one comes 4th, the final race determines who finishes on top.

The person in 4th place must have 7 points less than Jill if he is going to finish last (regardless of the scores in the last round).

The easiest way to do this is go through each option and see if the scores sum to 90. However, remember that 4th place gets 6 points in the last round so we need to take away 6 from each answer.

> Option E: 23 – If 4th place has 23 in round 10, they have 17 in round 9. Thus, Jill has 24 in round 9 and the rest have 31 each. This sums to 103. [Too high]
> Option D: 21 – If 4th place has 21 in round 10, they have 15 in round 9. Thus, Jill has 22 in round 9 and the rest have 29 each. This sums to 95. [Too high]
> Option C: 19 – If 4th place has 19 in round 10, they have 13 in round 9. Thus, Jill has 20 in round 9 and the rest have 27 each. This sums to 87. [Close enough!]

Question 32: A

This question can be worked out relatively quickly without determining exact values. There were 7000 people killed out of 2.3 million vehicles in 1930, and 3180 people killed out of 27 million today. There are roughly half the people killed for 10 times the number of vehicles, which gives a fraction of 1/20, or 0.04 times as much.

Question 33: D

It is important to read exactly what the question is asking you here. It wants reasons that are *not already in the text* which strengthen the case for roads become safer.
> A and C don't mean that roads are safer; if anything, it could mean that accidents are being under-reported (as mentioned in the article).
> B and E are valid points but are mentioned in the article already.
> D is a reasonable answer and gives us more of a reason to trust figures given in the article.

Question 34: C

This is probably the easiest question on the paper, and requires you to work out 40% of 319928. As the answer is wanted to the nearest 1000 anyway, 40% of 320000 is a reasonable calculation, which is 128000.

Question 35: A

> Although a very strong statement, it is the only answer that is plausible based on elimination and accounts for the discrepancy in the results.
> B is irrelevant, as roads being safer is unrelated to the discrepancy.
> C would mean that hospital admissions decrease, but they remain unchanged.
> D would mean the DfT figures should be higher than hospital figures.
> E would again make DfT figures higher than the hospital.

END OF SECTION

Section 2

Question 1: F
Homeostasis is defined as the maintenance of constant internal conditions. Homeostatic responses occur whether a factor rises or reduces, and internal body conditions can be affected by changes in variables inside our body (e.g. blood glucose levels) or changes in variables in the environment (e.g. temperature). Thus, all the statements could result in a homeostatic response.

Question 2: D
Atomic mass of bromobutane $= (12x4) + (9x1) + 80 = 137g/mol$
Atomic mass of butanol $= (12x4) + (10x1) + 16 = 74g/mol$
Since the molar ratio between bromobutane and butanol is 1:1, we can form: $\dfrac{2.74}{137} = \dfrac{x}{74}$ where x is the theoretical yield.

Rearranging gives: $x = \dfrac{2.74 x 74}{137} \dfrac{3 x 70}{140}$

$x = 1.5g$.
The actual yield is 1.1g. Therefore, $percentage yield = \dfrac{1.1}{1.5} x100 = 73.3\%$

Note that because we rounded earlier on to make the maths easier, the answer isn't exactly 75%. This, is fine because the options are far enough apart to make **D** the only obvious answer. Remember, to **look at the options first to see how freely you can round numbers.**

Question 3: B
The first step is α decay, as 2 protons are lost, giving R-2. This means 2 neutrons are also lost, meaning the atomic mass is decreased by 4.
The second step is β decay, so a neutron changes into a proton (plus an electron). This leaves the atomic mass unchanged as seen and the atomic number increases by 1. Thus, $P = N - 4$ and $Q = R - 1$

Question 4: A
There is no quick way to do this. Shaded Area $=$
$Largest Circle + 2nd largest circle - 3rd Largest Circle - Smallest Circle$
$= \pi\left(\dfrac{4d}{2}\right)^2 + \pi\left(\dfrac{2d}{2}\right)^2 - \pi\left(\dfrac{3d}{2}\right)^2 - \pi\left(\dfrac{d}{2}\right)^2$

$= \pi[4d^2 + d^2 - \dfrac{9d^2}{4} - \dfrac{d^2}{4}]$

$$= \pi[5d^2 + -\frac{10d^2}{4}]$$

$$= \pi d^2[5 - 2.5]$$

$$= \frac{5}{2}\pi d^2$$

Question 5: B
1. Nicotine acts at the nicotinic acetylcholine receptors in the brain, leading to addiction.
2. Bronchitis is an infection of the bronchi, which can be caused by smoking and the bronchi is what area 2 points to.
3. Emphysema is a disease causing damage to the alveoli in the lungs, making you short of breath, and can be caused by smoking.
4. Carbon monoxide can enter your blood stream via the alveoli due to the effects of smoking.

Question 6: C
Lecithin is an emulsifier which has a hydrophilic head forming bonds with water and a hydrophobic tail forming bonds with oil, to prevent separation.

Question 7: F
None of the radiation is stopped by the paper, suggesting there is no α radiation. Some of the radiation is stopped by aluminium, but not all of it, suggesting the presence of β and γ radiation.

NB: Don't confuse yourself by bringing background radiation into this – the question strongly implies that it's not relevant here e.g. detector is **close** to the radioactive source.

Question 8: E
Remember to take a step by step approach when rearranging formulae:

$$G = 5 + \sqrt{7(9-R)^2 + 9}$$

$$G - 5 = \sqrt{7(9-R)^2 + 9}$$

$$(G - 5)^2 = 7(9-R)^2 + 9$$

$$\frac{(G-5)^2 - 9}{7} = (9-R)^2$$

$$9 - R = \sqrt{\frac{(G-5)^2 - 9}{7}}$$

$$R = 9 - \sqrt{\frac{(G-5)^2 - 9}{7}}$$

Question 9: A
➤ The patient will no longer be able to sense pain if these neurons cannot detect stimuli normally causing pain.
➤ Statement 1 must be correct as it is involved in each answer. There would be no reflex response if the neuron does not sense any pain.
➤ Statement 2 is correct. If there is a visual stimulus, such as a pin prick coming towards you, then you would still move away based on vision alone.
➤ Statement 3 and 4 suggest that the patient can sense the pain but this is incorrect.

Question 10: D
It is easier to use an elimination method rather than trying to balance this equation manually. Start by balancing for Phosphorous, as it has relatively simple values in the equation. The quickest way to do this is via algebra (for more information, see the Chemistry chapter in *The Ultimate BMAT Guide*).

For Phosphorous: $A + B = 3C$;
Only Options C + D fulfil this equation. Thus, we can eliminate, A, B + E.
Next, for Hydrogen: $2A + B = 2D$; Only D fulfil this equation.

Question 11: D
For work to be done, a force must act in a parallel direction to the object.
1. The person sat on the chair hasn't moved so no work has been done.
2. The force is acting perpendicular to the direction of motion. Thus, whilst work is being done to move the barrow, $Work done \neq Fd$.
3. d represents the direction in which work is being done so $Work done = Fd$

Question 12: E

$$= \sqrt[3]{\frac{2x10^5}{\left(5x10^{-3}\right)^2}} - \sqrt{4x10^3 - 4x10^2}$$

$$= \sqrt[3]{\frac{2x10^5}{25x10^{-6}}} - \sqrt{4000 - 400}$$

$$= \sqrt[3]{\frac{2x10^5}{2.5x10^{-5}}} - \sqrt{3600}$$

$$= \sqrt[3]{0.8x10^{10}} - 60 = \sqrt[3]{8x10^9} - 60$$

$$= 2x10^3 - 60$$

$$= 2000 - 60$$

$= 1940$

Question 13: E

Answer 1 could be an explanation as the antibiotic discs Q and R have very similar effects on the bacterial colonies. Answer 2 is unrelated to the question and the fact that the antibiotic is working suggests there is little to no resistance. Answer 3 is potentially correct as this is where the distance up to which the bacteria are destroyed.

Question 14: F

As all of the possible formulae of azurite have 3 copper atoms, we know the stoichiometry of the reaction is 2 of one of the reagents and 1 of the other. We can test both of these combinations.

$2CuCO_3 + Cu(OH)_2$ à $Cu_3C_2H_2O_8$ which is as a possible answer.

$CuCO_3 + 2Cu(OH)_2$ à $Cu_3CH_4O_7$ which is not a possible answer.

Question 15: B

$Wavespeed = frequency x wavelength$

$f = \dfrac{3x10^8}{0.12}$, so f= 2.5 x 10⁹ Hz

As frequency stays constant, wavelength $= \dfrac{2.0x10^8}{2.5x10^9} = 0.08m = 8cm$

Question 16: C

There are several ways of doing this question. One of the simples is to form additional triangles by adding a point on the line MB.

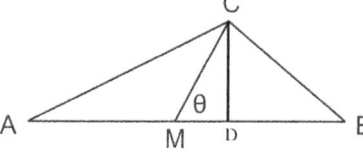

$Tan(x) = \dfrac{opposite}{adjacent}$ and since:

➢ Tan B= 2/3 à CD = 2 and DB = 3.

➢ Tan A = 1/6 à Since, CD is 2, $AD = 2x6 = 12$

➢ $AB = AD + DB = 12 + 3 = 15$

Then, looking at right angled triangle CMD, we know the opposite length is 2 and the adjacent length can be calculated as follows:

Since, M is the midpoint, $MD = 7.5 - DB = 4.5$

Therefore $Tan\theta = \dfrac{2}{4.5} = \dfrac{4}{9}$

Question 17: C

It is helpful to write out the relationship described:

Alcohol à ADH decreases à Dilute Urine produced. Thus, we can conclude that ADH concentrates urine.

1 is correct as all hormones travel in the bloodstream. There is a negative correlation between dilute urine production and ADH levels, rendering 2 and 3 incorrect. 4 is correct as increased formation of dilute urine means more water is lost and dehydration may occur.

Question 18: D

This requires you to have memorised the reactivity series. Zinc, and thus vanadium, are below Chlorine, Sodium, aluminium and magnesium in the reactivity series so they can be displaced by the more reactive elements. However, Zinc and vanadium are above iron in the reactivity series. Thus, the less reactive iron will not be able to displace the more reactive vanadium from a compound.

Question 19: D

Consider each factor in turn:

➤ Total resistance: The circuit changes from parallel to a series which have a higher overall resistance.

➤ Ammeter 1 measures overall current. Since, total resistance has increased, and the voltage is the same, the total current must decrease in accordance with Ohm's Law ($V = IR$).

➤ Ammeter 2 was measuring the current in a branch. Since, the circuit is now in series, the current no longer 'splits' at branches. Thus, the entire current flows through ammeter 2. Therefore the current flowing through this ammeter will increase.

Question 20: B

The balls are arranged to give the smallest possible probability for the player to win. Thus, the arrangement is:

➤ Bag 1: 2 red and 2 yellow

➤ Bag 2: 2 red, 1 yellow and 1 blue

There are 3 ways to win, each with equal probability:

➤ 2 yellows from bag 1

➤ 2 reds from bag 1

➤ 2 reds from bag 2

The probability of any choosing the correct bag = ½

Thus, the probability of picking the above permutations is given by:

$$= \frac{1}{2} x \frac{2}{4} x \frac{1}{3} = \frac{1}{12}$$

Since, there are 3 ways of winning, the probability of winning $= \frac{1}{12} x 3 = \frac{1}{4}$

Question 21: D

Statement 1 is wrong, as this does the opposite of explaining why there are less recessive phenotypes than expected. The other 2 reasons are correct and are fundamental ideas in scientific research (we need large sample sizes to reduce the effect of chance).

Question 22: B

This is easier than it looks. Remember that Helium is an inert gas so HeOH is not a plausible product. Tritium beta decays to a single Helium atom. Thus, Let T represent both Helium and Tritium in the equations below:

HTO à $H_2O + O_2 + T$ or   HTO à $H_2O + H_2 + T$

The first equation can be balanced as: 4HTO à $2H_2O + O_2 + 4T$ but the second equation cannot be balanced. Thus, the only possible products are those shown by option 2.

Question 23: D

$$Loss\,in\,E_p = mg\,\Delta h = 100x10x100 = 10^5 J$$

Since the cyclist descends 100m vertically, and for every 1m descended 10m is travelled along the road, the cyclist travels 1000m along the road.

Since Work is being done by the cyclist: Work Done = Force x Distance

Therefore, $Force = \dfrac{10^5}{10^3} = 10^2 N$

Since the cyclist is travelling at constant velocity, the resultant force must = 0. Thus: Resistive Force = Force due to weight = 100 N.

Question 24: A

This is a tough question:

➢ Let the cost of wood be y, and the cost of metal 3y
➢ Let the quantity of metal used be m_1, which is proportional to d
➢ Let the quantity of wood used be w_1, which is proportional to d^2
➢ Total Cost=3y x m_1+ y x w_1

Now we have 2d:

$m_2 = 2d = 2m_1$

$w_2 = (2d)^2 = 4d^2 = 4w_1$

3(total cost) = 3y x m_2 + y x w_2 = 6y x m_1+ 4y x w_1

Substitute for total cost: 3(3y x m_1 + y x w_1) = 6y x m_1 + 4y x w_1

$9m_1 + 3w_1 = 6m_1 + 4w_1$

$3m_1 = w_1$

Percentage of metal = $m_1/(m_1+w_1) = ¼ = 25\%$

Question 25: E

It is easiest to work backwards in each case.

Let's call the dominant allele A and the recessive allele a. Remember we are looking for the **minimum number**. When only U is recessive (aa), S and T must be heterozygous (Aa). If one was dominant, then they would not be able to produce offspring with the recessive condition.

R can be AA. Only one of P or Q must be Aa so that S is also heterozygous, giving a total of 3. When R is also recessive, P and Q must be heterozygous, along with S and T, giving a total of 4 heterozygous individuals.

Question 26: E

$C_2H_4 + H_2$ à C_2H_6

The pressure will initially increase due to the increase in temperature. However, the final pressure will be ½ of the initial pressure because:

➢ Pressure is determined the number of moles of a gas present and
➢ The products have ½ the number of moles as the reactants.

Question 27: G

➢ Statement P is wrong as the speed of sound is constant in air (330 m/s).
➢ Q is wrong because the amplitude would be half of the distance between X and Y (2.5 mm)
➢ R is wrong because we cannot comment on wavelength with the available data.
➢ Frequency $= \dfrac{1}{0.2 x 10^{-3}} = 1,000 x 5 = 5 k Hz.$
➢ Thus, only statement S is correct.

END OF SECTION

SECTION THREE

Section 3

"Doubt is not a pleasant condition, but certainty is absurd." (Voltaire)

> Voltaire suggests that whilst questioning something can be a very daunting feeling it is better than merely accepting something as certain. This statement therefore encapsulates the concept of science, where every idea and theory can be challenged and questioned. Many theories that have previously been accepted as 'truth' in the past are later falsified and revised. Doubt is at least a logical position where one can look for more answers and evidence.

> It can be argued that some things are 'certain' and are not necessarily absurd. At school we are taught that it is certain that the sun will rise tomorrow, and there has never been evidence to suggest otherwise. Of course, there is the miniscule possibility of a cataclysmic event, which would have to consist of something beyond our current knowledge of physics. However, does this factor mean it is 'absurd' to declare the sun rising as a certainty? Other things that seem certain include the fact that we are all currently living, and that somebody who is deceased will not come back to life.

> Good statement to promote scientific, rational and logical thinking scientific, but absurd may be too strong a word.

"There is something attractive about people who don't regard their own health and longevity as the most important things in the world." (Alexander Chancellor)

> This statement describes admiration for those who are unselfish and consider others needs as much as theirs. The chancellor condemns living egocentrically, whereby one is concerned only for prolonging their life and well-being.

> It can be argued that one's own health and longevity is more important than anything else; ultimately we are biological creatures who must undergo survival of the fittest in the evolutionary process of natural selection and thus our main aim is to preserve our genetic information, meaning our fitness is more important than other's fitness. We must compete with others and this involves placing ourselves above others. If we were to ignore this self-worth and put others above us, then we may also end up suffering. We only live once, and in that sense one's health and life can be regarded as highly precious (as its virtually irreplaceable) and therefore it should have the highest worth other others or material possessions.

> It is very humanitarian to consider other people's health and longevity; this can be through religious influences, or through 'humanist' principles. These argue that as a human race we should value each other's survival as a whole; that is perhaps a factor why we have progressed through the ages and seen this openness gradually accepted as a social norm today. Altruistic behaviour, empathy and many other traits based on selflessness are arguably what make us 'human'.

The scientist is not someone who gives the right answers but one who asks the right questions.

➢ The statement addresses the argument that science is not just about reading textbooks, memorizing info and regurgitating it when necessary; it is instead about asking the pertinent questions that allow scientific advancement.

➢ Scientists must be comfortable with the unknown to allow progression rather than needing answers to everything.

➢ A scientist cannot formulate satisfactory answers without satisfactory questions; a fundamental principle of scientific research is that a hypothesis, derived from a scientific question, must be present before any experimentation takes place.

➢ Science is about thinking "How does that work", or "why does this happen", and then trying to answer that question. Some of the most exciting science discoveries would never have happened, without that initial spark of inspiration from an inquisitive question. If Newton hadn't asked himself how the apple came to fall to Earth, or Darwin hadn't asked why the mockingbirds on different islands were separate species, could they possibly have found the answers to these questions?

➢ Insightful questions can challenge accepted models, and turn the way we think about a concept on its head. However, you still need a curious, inquisitive mind to come up with the right answers.

➢ Questions without answers are often frustrating and undesirable, suggesting the answer is at least as important as the question. Indeed, neuroscientists studying consciousness focus on the 'easy problems' which can be viably studied and avoid the 'hard problems' for which we do not even know how to approach to determine an answer.

➢ A scientific theory is empirical and is therefore always open to falsification. Accepted beliefs and conventions are changeable in science; what we believe to be true now could easily be disproved in 100 years, 50 years, or tomorrow. Inspiration for progression can come in several ways. It can come from realising that the old questions are no longer working, highlighting the importance of scientific questions. Or, it can come from thinking of new ways to approach old questions, and this represents innovation with the answer rather than the question

> Einstein claimed "I have no special talents, I am just passionately curious."

"... Dolphins are very intelligent and so similar to humans that they are worthy of a special ethical status: that of 'non-human persons'."

> Dolphins have distinct personalities, self-awareness, forward thinking, complex social structures, empathy, and many other 'higher' functions we previously only attributed to humans. The statement suggests that this should lead to the, having an ethical status of 'non-human persons' which will give them a legally enforceable right to life.

> Animals are generally all bound by equal animal rights, whereas humans are bound by equal human rights, and within these groups we do not differentiate for intelligence. Why should there be an exception for dolphins?

> We have no concept of what being a dolphin is like, as they live in a completely different environment and have different lifestyles. We currently mistreat them and should they not be protected from exploitation?

> Intelligence is an extraordinary attribute, and the fact that they are self-aware and are likely to experience similar emotions in a similar way to us means it appears unethical to use them for our entertainment or kill them for food, suggesting they deserve these rights.

> Are there many downsides to giving dolphins rights? Most people don't aim to kill them either deliberately or inadvertently, and there isn't much to lose. If they are sentient beings whose intelligence warrants such rights then it seems like a rational idea. All life is sacred, but arguably those with higher levels of consciousness deserve more respect and more protection.

> If an animal is more intelligence than another should it receive greater treatment? The notion because x is smarter than y then x should not be killed brings many ethical implications along with it. Should more intelligent humans have better rights than less intelligent humans? (Or you could argue that they already do, through privilege). Again, it depends how one defines intelligence - 'don't judge a fish by its ability to climb a tree.'

➣ "Intelligent" behaviour of various kinds is found in many animals and when we measure intelligence, we do so according to a human (and culturally specific) norm. Even in testing human intelligence, there is controversy over these issues. Why should intelligence be the standard for conferring rights? Does this mean that mentally handicapped humans or those suffering from dementia should be denied rights? Then, there is a question as to whether these rights are to be extended to all cetaceans or only the most intelligent ones.

➣ One can support the protection of animals, but intelligence appears to be a rigid standard to use in order to decide which animals deserve what protection.

END OF PAPER

2013

Section 1

Question 1: A

This question can be worked out sequentially using the information given. Carla isn't working on Monday, which means Bob and Amy must be. That fills Bob quota of 3 days in the week. This means Carla and Amy must be working on Wednesday and Thursday. Amy cannot also work on Tuesday, as that would make it 4 consecutive days, so Carla must work on Tuesday too.

Question 2: C

- ➢ A is a very bold statement and probably too strong to even be considered. The passage doesn't say that life can't exist on Kepler-22b and in fact even suggests that its new reclassification as uninhabitable may be inaccurate.
- ➢ B suggests the opposite of the background we are given. Cosmologists now suggest that less planets are habitable than previously thought.
- ➢ C summarises a main conclusion of the passage and is thus the best answer. The passage gives the example of Earth; that it is close to being outside the habitable zone but is robustly life-friendly, doubting the accuracy of the criteria.
- ➢ D cannot be inferred from this information alone. The passage doesn't describe a link between clouds and Kepler-22b.

Question 3: C

There are 6 combinations, and each one can be tested by determining the number of days between birthdays. If this equals a multiple of 7 then their birthdays are always on the same day of the week. 281 - 218 = 63, so Adam and Tara have their birthdays on the same day of the week every year.

Question 4: C

The main conclusion of the argument is easy to spot in this argument, as it is at the end of the passage and begins with the word 'therefore.'

- ➢ A, B and D are points which are mentioned in the text, but only as background information and they do not constitute the conclusion of the passage.
- ➢ C paraphrases the conclusion that "*the secret to losing weight is painfully simple - do more and/or eat less*" and is thus the best answer.
- ➢ E is incorrect as the conclusion also describes that eating less can lead to calorie burn.

Question 5: D

Jason sold y Spruggles on day 1, and 2y on day 2. They cost £12 on day 1 and £9 on day 2, and he made £342 more on day 2. Thus y x 12 + 342 = 2y x 9. We want 3y (how many were sold altogether).

$18y = 12y + 342$

$6y = 342$

$3y = 171$

Question 6: C

The main point of the Clovis-First theory is that the Clovis were *the first inhabitants* of the Americas.

C is the only answer that would seriously challenge this point, as it has a specific time linked to it. The Clovis first theory suggests that they arrived at -11500 BC, and if there was a human settlement present 500 years before this time then this disproves the theory.

The other answers all link to the background information given, and could all be legitimate in a 'weaken' question, but none others seriously challenge that the Clovis were the first inhabitants.

Question 7: A

➢ Although elimination may seem quite a long process on the surface, it can be done rather quickly.

➢ Simon has 5 letters in his name so is limited to Hyde and Rush, and cannot be Rush because of the letter s. **Simon Hyde**

➢ Liam has 4 letters in his name so is limited to Doyle, Floyd and Shore, and must be Shore because of the letter l. **Liam Shore**

➢ Dylan has 5 letters in his name and must thus be Rush. **Dylan Rush**

➢ Eric must be Doyle or Floyd. It cannot be Doyle due to the letter e. **Eric Floyd.** Thus Ian's surname must be Doyle. **Ian Doyle**

Question 8: D

D is clearly the correct answer, especially given that the question tells you that it is a sarcastic comment. If you find it hard to spot sarcasm, then we can rule out B and C as the comment links to the quote about children rather than the other 2, and the sarcasm of 'no' means we should agree with whatever the quote says, which is paraphrased in D.

Question 9: A
Answer A basically paraphrases this 'evidence' and is thus the correct answer. The statement does not relate to what wealth should bring, or anything about children. D assumes a causality which is not necessarily suggested by the statement.

Question 10: D
1. Kahneman suggests that the better you are at the job, the more time you must invest in it. However, this does not necessarily imply that people who work shorter hours will give more time to their children - they may use this 'extra' time in other ways.
2. The transcript talks about not getting happier as we get richer over a certain level. However, it does not suggest that wealth under this level will not cause stress.

Question 11: B
Anecdotal evidence is evidence based on personal accounts rather than facts or research, which this story clearly is. It is not necessarily conclusive without facts to back it up, there are no statistics and it is relevant. We can argue that it is not hearsay as it is said that she is intimately involved with the family she describes.

Question 12: B
BEWARE that the symbol for Mercury and the symbol for Venus/Copper look very similar.
We can use the process of elimination here.
We can start with the first card, and at the top. There is only 1 equivalent to moon, which is silver on card 4, but the second item is different, so we can rule out cards 1 and 4 for having a pair.
The second card has 3 equivalents for the top item - cards 6, 7 and 8. The second item is only equivalent for card 7, and the last item for cards 2 and 7 are different, thus we can rule out all these cards as having a pair.
We are left with cards 3 and 5, and we can see that these are equivalent. Thus we have 1 pair in total.

Question 13: D
The main conclusion of the argument is "*In the interests of providing the most desirable outcomes, it is clear that placebos should be used as a treatment offered by the NHS.*" Thus, if treatments (such as placebos) ensure better outcomes, they should be used, which is paraphrased in D.
A doesn't necessarily support the argument, as you do not know whether the placebo will work. B, C and E are unrelated to the fundamental point of the argument.

Question 14: B

We can start by ruling out 8 and 5, as this would break the alphabetical order rule. Let's call the missing digits x and y. From the information given in the text, we know that $4 + 0 + x + y = 8 +$ number of letters in x + number of letters in y. So $x + y = 4 +$ number of letters in x and y.

Testing this rule out gives the exclusive answer of $x + y$ being 9 and 2. Here, it is important to re-read the question and make sure you give the number of letters that make up these digits, which is 7.

Question 15: B

A and C actually strengthen the argument as they back up some of the points made in the passage. D is a point against the argument, but doesn't weaken it, and is merely a statement saying the opposite of the passage. B is clearly the best answer as it directly contradicts the point that *"sport is what people do to counter the stress and pressures of work"* which is a key point in the author's argument that the growth of extreme sports is puzzling.

Question 16: C

- ➤ It is useful to quickly jot down the first letter of each month on a rough sheet of paper. J F M A M J J A S O N D. You can then determine which months the birthdays can occur on, along with the number of the month in the year.
- ➤ Jenny's and Alice's birthdays are 2 months apart - you can determine that this is only possible if Jenny's birthday is in June. It can't be in January or July because there would be no month 2 months away beginning with "A". Alice's birthday could be in August or April.
- ➤ Alice's and Michael's birthdays are 5 months apart - you can determine that this is only possible if Alice's birthday is in August and Michael's is in March, using the same logic as above. Thus Jenny's birthday is in June, Michael's is in March, making them 3 months apart.

Question 17: D

This argument suggests that age makes us lack sleep and age makes us have impaired memory, so the lack of sleep must cause the impaired memory. This is an error of reasoning.

1 and 3 highlight different ways that these ideas may be connected, aside from lack of sleep causing impaired memory, highlighting weaknesses in the error of reasoning. 2 is unrelated to this error of reasoning and doesn't weaken the argument.

Question 18: B

Start by writing all the square numbers between 1 and 60. The month must be 09, the day can be between 1-30, the hour can be between 1-24 and the minute can be between 1-60.

There are 4 possible days: 1, 4, 16, 25. If we start with day 01, then there are 8 times: 4:16, 4:25, 4:36, 4:49, 16:04, 16:25, 16:36 and 16:49. There will be the same number of times for days 4 and 16, as you can have 2 different hours and 4 times per hour without including the same square number, giving 24 times from these particular days. However, for day 25, there are more possible days, as you can have 3 different hours: 1, 4 and 16. These have 4 times per hour each, giving 12 times in total from this day. 24 + 12 = 36.

Question 19: B

There is no possible way that X can be green. The bottom left region must be green; it cannot be blue, yellow or red as there would be an edge with the same colour on both sides. The region to the top right of X can be red or yellow. When it is red, X can be yellow or blue. When it is yellow, X can be red or blue. Thus the region can be yellow, blue or red.

Question 20: C

If this circle was smaller than a square, and contained within a square, it could be the opposite colour to the square and no rules would be broken. If it was not contained within a square, or larger than a square, then it would have to be a different colour to the black and white to prevent any edge having the same colour on both sides.

Question 21: A

This is probably best done by trial and error. Try using 3 lines in many different combinations, and you will eventually see that 2 colours will always be sufficient, as a segment will never share an edge with more than 2 other segments, both of which can be the other colour.

Question 22: B

We can think of the top and bottom as 2 separate circles (or any shape) with 5 separate segments. If we look at the circles individually, we can see that 2 colours cannot suffice, as there would have to be 2 adjacent. 3 colours suffice. When we superimpose this on another circle, 3 colours are sufficient to never have 2 adjacent faces the same colour.

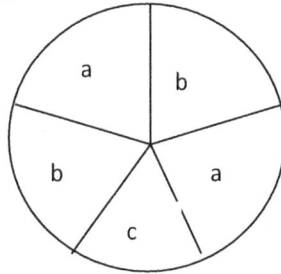

Question 23: D

Types of tile:

> Fully black
> ½ black
> ¼ black
> ¾ black

> Black line outlines ¼
> Black line outlines ½

2 X Black line outlines ½, ¼ black - this may be the one that people miss, as there are 2 forms of this shape and one cannot be rotated to form the other. If in doubt, take a rough piece of paper, draw the shape and try rotating it to see whether the tiles are equivalent.

Question 24: B

The main conclusion of this article is that *"to reduce the harm done by alcohol, it is vital to reduce consumption."* The author argues that one of the best ways to do this is to make alcohol more expensive. Answer B suggests that cheaper prices have led to more consumption of alcohol, backing up the point that alcohol consumption is based on price.

Answer A is irrelevant to the point about reducing consumption and answers C and D do not strengthen the argument.

Question 25: B

> The clocks are 41 minutes apart. The hour change must between 19 and 20. Within the same hour there would be the same digit used, or with the same first hour digit. 23 to 00 cannot be used as the 0 is used twice and 09 to 10 also uses the 0 twice.

> **19:ab and 20:cd:** c cannot be 0, 1 or 2 as these numbers are already used. It cannot be 4 as cd could only be 40 or 41 (41 minutes apart), and the 0 and 1 digits have been used. Therefore, c must be 3, and a is 5.

> **19:5b and 20:3d:** b or d cannot be 1, 2, 3, 5 or 9 as these have been used. If b is 4, then d would have to be 5 which is not possible. b can be 6 or 7 and d can be 7 or 8.

> **19:56-19:57 and 20:37 and 20:38.** There is no 4 used here.

Question 26: A

There is no easy way to do this- if you struggle with spatial awareness then this would be extremely difficult. Number 5 makes contact with P followed by 7 onto Q, 4 onto R and 1 onto S.

Question 27: C

We know Al is married and Charles is unmarried. Beth could be married or unmarried. C is the correct statement, as one way or the other, there was someone married looking at someone unmarried.

Question 28: D

The argument is *against* the idea that children should be exposed to harsh realities from a young age. Only D supports this, whereas the others suggest the opposite.

Question 29: E

Again this was a difficult spatial awareness question and the only quick way to solve it would be to actually make the net in the exam. The rules don't explicitly state that you may not use scissors although you should certainly approve it with your exams officer before. If spatial awareness isn't your forte- this was certainly one question to skip.

Question 30: D

1 and 3 are fundamental principles of evolution, which can be assumed when the word evolution is used. The argument says *"this characteristic must have evolved because it gave human beings a better grip underwater"* and this would not have 'evolved' if it were not advantageous. 2 is true from our previous knowledge, but is irrelevant to the argument and does not need to be assumed at any point.

Question 31: A

> First write down all the remaining numbers between 3 and 12, and cross each one out when used.

- **Bottom row:** 10+12=22, so the other 2 numbers must be add up to 7 to make 29. This means they must be 3 and 4, although we do not yet know in which order.
- **Top row:** 5+9=14, so the other 2 numbers must add up to 15. This can only be made from 7 and 8, although we do not yet know in which order.
- **Right column:** 11 must be above the 6, and we require 12 more. This means top right must be 8 and bottom right must be 4. This makes the person opposite 9 as 3.

Question 32: B

If 1% of non-cannabis users in the sample develop psychosis, and cannabis users were 41% more likely to have psychosis, 1.41% of cannabis users in the sample will have psychosis. 20% of young people report using cannabis, which is 2000 people.
2000 x 0.0141 = 2 x 14.1 = 28.2 users.

Question 33: A

Let's call the probability of psychosis for reasons other than cannabis use y. 80% of the population have probability y of getting psychosis, whereas 20% of the population have probability y plus the extra 41%.

We thus have 1.41 x 0.2y + 0.8y as the probability of getting psychosis and the percentage of getting it through cannabis use is:

$$\frac{0.41x0.2y}{1.41x0.2y + 0.8y} = \frac{0.082}{1.08} \frac{0.08}{1.1}$$

This gives a percentage of slightly less than 8%, so A must be correct.

Question 34: B

The passage suggests that an increase in x (cannabis use) causes an increase in y (psychosis), whereas this answer provides an alternative link and suggests that y may also cause an increase in x.

A mentions age but this is not an alternative reason for the link. C suggests that the link may not be valid, which is irrelevant to what the question is asking. D is a point against an alternative link, suggesting more psychotic patients may have used cannabis than we think.

Question 35: C

Causal link is the key phrase here, and is a common theme in science and thus the BMAT. We need some evidence that A to B may be more than just a correlation.

➢ A may look tempting on the surface, but it again doesn't prove causation. There may be a separate causal factor which affects you when young or old that links to cannabis and psychosis, rather than the cannabis itself.

➢ B, if anything, is against a direct causal link between cannabis and psychosis, highlighting that other factors may be involved.

➢ C suggests a causal link, because an increase in X (cannabis strength) **caused** an increase in Y (psychosis).

➢ D is irrelevant to showing a causal link.

➢ E is irrelevant to showing a causal link.

END OF SECTION

Section 2

Question 1: H
Both the nervous system and the endocrine system are involved in homeostasis. Some of the messaging takes place using chemicals and they can receive and send messages to and from the brain.

Question 2: D
This refers to the reactivity series. A displacement reaction can take place if the element in the salt is lower down in the reactivity series than the element it is being reacted with. This only applies to 1 and 4, where Al and Zn and higher in the reactivity series than Pb and Cu respectively.

Question 3: D
Both 1 and 2 are correct in their ability to damage. However, infrared does not cause damage when penetrating matter.

Question 4: A

$$\frac{4.6x10^7 + 7x2x10^6}{4.6x10^7 - 2x2x10^6}$$

$$= \frac{4.6x10^7 + 14x10^6}{4.6x10^7 - 4x10^6}$$

$$= \frac{4.6x10^7 + 1.4x10^7}{4.6x10^7 - 0.4x10^7}$$

$$= \frac{6.0x10^7}{4.2x10^7}$$

$$= \frac{6}{4.2}$$

$$= \frac{60}{42}$$

$$= \frac{10}{7}$$

Question 5: F

Protease would break down proteins into amino acids; lipase would break down fats into fatty acids and therefore lower the pH of the solution. However, carbohydrase would function to break up the carbohydrates and would produce the non-acidic sugar products, therefore not lowering the pH.

Question 6: B

This reaction is in equilibrium, with the greater number of moles on the left hand side of the equation than the left. This means that an increase in pressure would push the equilibrium to the right, therefore producing more T product. In addition, since the forward reaction is exothermic, a lower temperature shifts the equilibrium towards the products. Catalysts have no effect on yield of product, just on reaction speed, and addition of more reactants would obviously increase the product yield.

Question 7: H

The switch being closed has turned the circuit from a series to parallel which therefore has a lower overall resistance. Since total voltage is unchanged, current must increase in accordance with V=IR. Thus P increases. With the switch open, the voltage is shared across both resistors but with it closed, the second resistor can be bypassed (short-circuited) by the new branch. This means that only the full voltage is shared by the first resistor only. Thus, Q increases and R decreases.

Question 8: F

$$4 - \frac{x^2(1 - 16x^2)}{(4x - 1)2x^3} \quad = \quad 4 - \frac{(1 - 16x^2)}{2x(4x - 1)}$$

Thus: $\dfrac{8x(4x - 1)}{2x(4x - 1)} - \dfrac{(1 - 4x)(1 + 4x)}{2x(4x - 1)}$

$$= \frac{8x(4x - 1)}{2x(4x - 1)} + \frac{(4x - 1)(4x + 1)}{2x(4x - 1)}$$

Thus: $\dfrac{8x}{2x} + \dfrac{(4x + 1)}{2x}$

$$= \frac{8x + 4x}{2x} + \frac{1}{2x}$$

$$= 6 + \frac{1}{2x}$$

Question 9: F

Sensory neurons are the longest types of neurons as they must travel all the way to the spinal cord. The relay neurons are the shortest because they are only present in the spinal cord.

Question 10: B

This involves the equation $2Na + 2H_2O \rightarrow H_2 + 2NaOH$. You can therefore work out the moles of sodium by using $Mass = moles \times M_r$:

$$Moles\,of\,Sodium = \frac{1.15}{23} = 0.5\,moles$$

Since the molar ratio between Sodium and hydrogen gas is 2:1, 0.25 moles of hydrogen are produced.

Therefore, Volume of Hydrogen $= 22.4 \times 0.25 = 5.6\,dm^3 = 560\,cm^3$.

Question 11: C

Remember that:

➢ Angle of incidence < Critical Angle: Light Reflected Back
➢ Angle of incidence = Critical Angle: Total Internal Reflection
➢ Angle of incidence > Critical Angle: Light leaves outside

Diagram 1 is has an angle below the critical angle. Therefore, total internal reflection does not occur and instead the light is reflected out. In diagram 2, the angle is greater than the critical angle. Therefore, total internal reflection does not occur and instead the light passes through.

Question 12: B

Label the corners of the square as A, B C and D and then see where they move in relation to the transformations performed. A reflection in the y axis therefore leads to the original orientation.

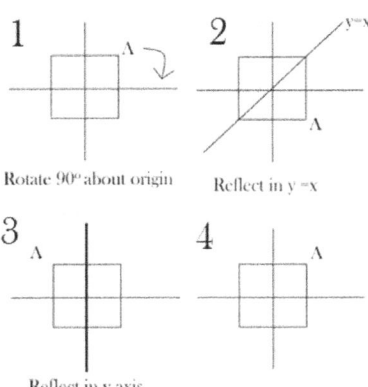

Question 13: C

The actual protein is not needed to produce it, as the intention is to allow the bacteria to produce the protein from the implanted DNA.

Question 14: A

In $MgCl_2$, the 2 valence electrons in Mg will each go to a chlorine atom, which will then mimic a filled orbital. The chloride atoms will both have the same electronic structure as argon, but when the Mg loses 2 electrons it will have the same electronic structure as neon, meaning the pair don't match.

Question 15: D

Don't get confused – this is actually easy since background radiation has been corrected for.

Source X has a half-life of 4.8 hours and thus has 5 half-lives in 24 hours.

$$Activity of X = 320 x 0.5^5 = 320 x \frac{1}{32} = 10$$

Source Y has a half-life of 8 hours and thus has 3 half-lives in 24 hours.

$$Activity of Y = 480 x 0.5^3 = 480 x \frac{1}{8} = 60$$

$$Total Activity = 60 + 10 = 70$$

Question 16: D

Start off by writing the relationships mathematically: $x z^2 and y \frac{1}{z^3}$

Now make the powers equivalent so we can substitute: $x^3 z^6 and y^2 \frac{1}{z^6}$

$$So y^2 \frac{1}{x^3} and x^3 \frac{1}{y^2}$$

Question 17: A

This question requires knowledge of somatic cell nuclear transfer. 2 is incorrect, because this procedure doesn't involve sperm cells. 4 is also incorrect, because the egg with the newly transferred nucleus must begin to divide, and not differentiate (point 1). The other 3 points are valid.

Question 18: E

NaOH + HCl à NaCl + H_2O

The atomic mass of NaOH = 23 + 16 + 1 = 40

Theoretical maximum of NaOH in sample: $\frac{1.2}{40} = 0.03$

Moles of NaOH in sample that react is given by $n = cV$:

$$\frac{50}{1000} x 0.5 = 0.025$$

Purity: $\frac{0.025}{0.03} = \frac{5}{6} = 83.3\%$

SECTION TWO

Question 19: D

Recall that Power $= IV = I^2R$. Since the resistors are in series, the overall current is given by: $I = \dfrac{V}{R1 + R2}$

Thus, Power $= (\dfrac{V}{R1 + R2})^2 R1 = \dfrac{V^2 R1}{(R1 + R2)^2}$

Question 20: D

Smallest Cube:

We have 5 faces of the smaller shape, which is 5 x 1= **5 cm²**

Middle Cube:

Where the small cube joins the middle cube, we have a right angled triangle with lengths x, x and 1. Using Pythagoras: $1^2 = x^2 + x^2 = 2x^2$

$x = \sqrt{\dfrac{1}{2}} = \dfrac{\sqrt{2}}{2}.$

Since the triangle makes up half the side, the total length of the side $=\sqrt{2}$

There are 4 faces fully uncovered and one face partially covered by the smaller shape.

Thus, the surface area $= 4x\sqrt{2}x\sqrt{2} = 8$

Surface area of top face $= \sqrt{2}x\sqrt{2}-1= 1$

Surface Area of 2nd layer $= 8 + 1= $ **9 cm²**

Largest Cube:

Using Pythagoras again: $\sqrt{2}^2 = x^2 + x^2 = 2x^2$

$2x^2 = 2$

Thus, $x = 1$. Since the triangle makes up half the side, the total length of the side $= 2$.

There are 5 faces fully uncovered and one face partially covered by the smaller shape.

Thus, the surface area $= 5x2x2 = 20$

Surface area of top face $= 2x2-2= 2$

Surface Area of 3rd layer $= 20 + 2= $ **22 cm²**

Total Surface Area: $5 + 9 + 22 = $ **36 cm²**

Question 21: E

The entire genome is found in every cell in the body, hence 1 and 2 are correct. Starch is broken down before it reaches the liver so 3 is incorrect.

Question 22: C

There are 2 atoms of Cr in the equation, so **d** must be 2. The equation must balance for charge, so **b** must be 8. Comparing **a** and **c** shows that these coefficients change the number of oxygens only and do not affect the number of carbons or hydrogens. Thus to have the correct number of hydrogens, **e** must be 4. **a** and **c** are 3, but this does not have to be deduced in this question.

Question 23: D

A. Rearrangement of $F = ma$

B. Rearrangement of $V = IR$

C. Rearrangement of $E_k = \dfrac{mv^2}{2}$

D. The relationship between wavelength and frequency is given by: $v = f$. If the y axis was wavelength, the axis should be $\dfrac{1}{f}$ i.e. the inverse of frequency (not a direct correlation).

E. Rearrangement of $Work Done = Force x Distance$

Question 24: C

We need to calculate the probability of either:

➢ 2 blue balls and 1 red ball

➢ 2 red balls and 1 blue ball

Each combination has 3 permutations (i.e. the first combination can be BBR or BRB or RBB).

Probability of 2 Blue Balls $= \dfrac{8}{10} x \dfrac{7}{9} x \dfrac{2}{8} x 3 = \dfrac{336}{720}$

Probability of 2 Red Balls $= \dfrac{2}{10} x \dfrac{1}{9} x \dfrac{8}{8} x 3 = \dfrac{48}{720}$

Total Probability $= \dfrac{48}{720} + \dfrac{336}{720}$

$\dfrac{384}{720} = \dfrac{8}{15}$

Question 25: C

Let's call the dominant allele A and the recessive allele a. We're looking for the proportion of Aa cats. 50% in the first cross, and 67% in the second (dead organisms don't contribute to a population).

	A	a
A	Aa ($\frac{1}{4}$)	aa ($\frac{1}{4}$)
A	Aa ($\frac{1}{4}$)	aa ($\frac{1}{4}$)
	A	a

A	AA (dead)	Aa ($\frac{1}{3}$)
a	Aa ($\frac{1}{3}$)	aa ($\frac{1}{3}$)

Question 26: B

3, then 6.

As a catalyst is not used up in the reaction, we can see that using 3 then 6 uses NO to speed up the reaction but then replenishes it at the end.

We can also see that a by-product which is not present in the net production, NO_2, is used up before the final products are formed.

Finally, the reagents used which are used up at SO_2 and $\frac{1}{2}$ O_2 as seen in the reaction, and SO_3 is the only net product generated.

Question 27: E

The kinetic energy is given by $\frac{mv^2}{2}$ i.e. $\frac{4v^2}{2} = 1800$.

Thus, $v = 30$ ms^{-1}

Using $F = ma$, the current acceleration is $= \frac{20}{4} = 5ms^{-2}$

Now calculate the velocity after 2 seconds of acceleration by the same force by using:
$v = u + at$: $v = 30 + 2x5 = 40$

Then calculate the final kinetic energy: $\frac{4x40^2}{2} = 3200$ J.

Finally, the extra kinetic energy is the difference between 3200 and 1800 = 1400 J

END OF SECTION

SECTION THREE

Section 3

"When you want to know how things really work, study them when they are coming apart." (William Gibson)

> This statement suggests that the function of a system is not fully represented when it is working smoothly, rather it is only when the system is put under stressful conditions that the intricacies and factors in the system can be fully appreciated. This concept can be appreciated from a tangible example of a working system, such as the internal structures in a clock. When certain cogs in the clock fall out or stop working, it is easy to identify their place in the overall system. This follows the suggestion by the phrase that a functioning system can mask certain important properties that the system possesses. A system 'coming apart' allows identification of different parts, their purposes and their importance with regards to the function of the whole system. This can be represented by the mutation of certain genes leading to defects, such as in the case of cystic fibrosis, the mutation in the chloride channel shows its vital involvement in the secretion of mucus. In addition, 'coming apart' can help identify the original function of the system, as it will presumably be unable to perform it under those conditions.

> This method for studying systems does however have flaws. If the entire representation of the system is based on the lack of function of the system, this means that in some cases, the original function of cannot be understood. The use of such a principle therefore relies heavily on background knowledge, as without some understanding of the system, its lack of function could mean very little. For example, a certain part of a computer can malfunction, leading to a complete breakdown; however, without understanding the basics of what each part in the computer provides to the function, there will be too many unknowns to really build up an understanding. Additionally, if more than one factor leads to the coming apart of the system, a more subtle function of a part could be masked by a less subtle function of another.

> This method also underestimates the complexity of the system and the number of factors that may be interacting. It also does not allow you to appreciate the system as a whole.

> Overall, this method could be applicable in a simple system that there is already basic knowledge in place. However, for a more complex system that includes the involvement of a number of parts, or a system that has yet to be investigated, it may not accurately represent all the interacting features.

Good surgeons should be encouraged to take on tough cases, not just safe, routine ones. Publishing an individual surgeon's mortality rates may have the opposite effect.

➤ Tough cases present a challenge to surgeons, as increased difficulty of the procedure leads to an increased risk of mortality. It is therefore suggested that due to this increased likelihood of mortality, doctors may be reluctant to take tough cases on if the records were public as their reputation would be somewhat tarnished if the operations were unsuccessful. Public exposure of surgical league tables could also prevent consent from certain patients for certain surgeons to carry out procedures. In particular, certain cases of high mortality rates in surgeons could show that the surgeon is more experienced as they have performed in situations of increased risk. The surgeon could also feel increased pressure in certain procedures, leading to potential negative outcomes. This league table could also undermine the expertise of both the GMC and the hospital, which must make regular reviews of their doctors to make sure that they are working to the best of their abilities. In addition, mortality rates give very little information about the situation in which the death took place and in a number of cases, it could have no reflection on the surgeon at all.

➤ Publishing mortality rates could also have a positive impact on surgeons. I suggested above that this could put the surgeons under increased pressure, however all doctors should feel a certain pressure as they have a responsibility to the patient. In the case of the surgeon, they hold patient's life in their hands and they should not forget that they are obligated to perform to the best of their ability. Slightly contrastingly, a league table should have no impact on the performance of a doctor, as a doctor must always act with the patient's best interest at heart, rather than worrying about their reputation. Patients also have a right to know the performance record of a doctor, as they are putting their welfare into their hands, and therefore have a right to know all the factors and risks involved in making such a decision, including their surgeon.

➤ To use such a league table for the improvement of surgical performance would be extremely beneficial; however it is unlikely that this would be the case. It is more likely that there will be a negative impact on surgical performance, or even the decision to perform the surgery in the first place. In conclusion it is probably more beneficial for both the surgeon and the patient that the league table be kept private, as it enables the doctors to act as they see fit, potentially saving more lives due to the undertaking of riskier but more beneficial operations.

"Ignorance more frequently begets confidence than does knowledge: it is those who know little, and not those who know much, who so positively assert that this or that problem will never be solved by science." (Charles Darwin)

➢ Darwin is suggesting that people who know very little about science are very confident that they know the limits of the field and therefore do not think it is able to make progress in certain areas. This can be valid idea in certain respects as little knowledge of a subject can cause a person to think they know the important aspects of a certain field. It might however actually be the case that the field has much more complexities that can offer very exciting potential developments, something which could be overlooked by an ignorant person.

➢ This concept can be represented by a self-diagnosis made by a patient online, they are only being exposed to very superficial (and potentially incorrect) areas of the field and this can lead them to incorrect conclusions.

➢ On the contrary this concept does not always apply. When looking at research environments, it is possible for a very knowledgeable researcher to have studied the subject for such an extended period of time that their sense of the bigger picture becomes clouded. This could mean that an ignorant person is then able to come and have a different take on the problem, as they have not developed the same mind-set of the knowledgeable researcher and they are less aware of possible limitations of the field, able to look 'outside the box'.

➢ This can be compared to a partnership between an engineer and a biologist in the development of medical equipment, the engineer might not know very much about biology, they are however able to give a different outlook on the problem. Similarly a scientist very knowledgeable in a field may not be able to accept that the field may be unable to progress, something that an ignorant person may be able to notice. There is also the possibility that an ignorant person may assume that science has not limits, which can be helpful and detrimental depending on the situation.

➢ Overall, this attitude does have some truth, I find however that it is cynical and a generalisation. It does not take into account that it is new and possibly initially ignorant minds that are pushing the boundaries of science, allowing it progress at a rapid pace.

In a world where we struggle to feed an ever-expanding human population, owning pets cannot be justified.

- This phrase suggests that the expense of owning a pet is unnecessary, rather the resources used to support a pet should be used to help support the over-expanding population. This argument is based on a number of assumptions and I will attempt to sort through them here.
- On one hand, it is true that the population is 'over-expanding' and we have a moral obligation to support those in need. It is also true that ownership of a pet requires a lot of resources. The pet must be fed, watered and housed appropriately. This therefore suggests that the owner must have food and money available for this particular purpose. One could argue that the money spent on the pet and the food that it consumes, could be better used elsewhere. If the resources used to support the pet were dedicated to support the needs of the expanding population, it is possible that a significant positive contribution to the cause could be made. In addition, one could argue that some expensive and exotic pets are an unnecessary luxury and too indulgent.
- On the other hand, the above statement assumes that the resources and food supplied to pets could be better used elsewhere. Owning a pet is an individual's decision, a choice to spend their money how they please. There is also no guarantee that even if these owners did not own a pet they would spend the equivalent amount supporting those in need, they might instead buy something equivalently recreational.
- An extrapolation of the above statement might lead one to say "why don't we restrict television sales and other such luxuries as the funds could be better used elsewhere?" As further support against this statement, it is important to consider the importance of pet ownership, such as the life-saving duties of guide dogs, likely to be considered a worthwhile expense. In addition, ownership of pets in some cases can reduce the wastage due to their consumption of leftover food, which would have been otherwise discarded.
- Additionally, the money spent on pets can be a form of support for the economy. A stronger economy allows the government to provide more assistance to those in need.
- In conclusion, we have a moral obligation to help those in need, however, pet ownership and lack of resources for an expanding population are not necessarily correlated, as the ownership cannot account the a massive resource deficit. Making steps to prevent food wastage or encouraging charitable donations may be a more worthwhile venture.

END OF PAPER

2014

Official Worked Solutions for the 2014 paper are freely available online at **www.uniadmissions.co.uk/bmat-past-papers**. This link will take you to a page where you can download ALL past paper as well as the 2014 solutions (you will have to provide your email for the download link).

Alternatively, you can download the papers and 2014 solutions from the link here: **https://bit.ly/2MGipmM**

2015

Section 1

Question 1: D
Plotting the information:
Stuart > Ruth > Margaret
Tim > Adrian?
We don't know where Adrian sits in relation to Margaret, but we do know that Adrian is shorter than Tim, Ruth and Stuart. So Adrian is shorter than Ruth and Stuart but not necessarily Margaret.

Question 2: E
E- is the overall conclusion from the passage as it states *" three quarters of all infections recorded last year were in people from deprived areas...and born outside"*, thus only a quarter were from more affluent populations and born in the UK.

A may be true but is a posed as a potential reason to account for the weakened immune systems that may again be the cause of the increased incidence of TB in deprived areas, so it is not a conclusion. B,C and D may again be true but are not conclusions, they are possible reasons for the overall conclusion that TB incidence has increased but in not in UK born affluent populations.

Question 3: A
The readings show the end of month readings so to find the greatest difference between September 1ˢᵗ and November 30ᵗʰ subtract the November readings from August (as August reading is end of the month, hence the value for September 1ˢᵗ).

	August	November	Difference
Red	68 240	78 853	**10 613**
Orange	64 425	73 684	9 259
Yellow	71 302	81 163	9 861
Green	64 827	75 146	10 319
Blue	73 959	83 392	9 433
Indigo	68 623	78 229	9 606
Violet	63 088	72 826	9 738

The red van has the biggest difference so the answer is A.

Question 4: A

A if true would best express a flaw in the overall conclusion of the passage that physical attractiveness correlates with sporting performance, as it highlights the failure of the passage to account for other potential contributing factors to sporting success.

B is not true as an objective measurement has been taken using performance in a cycling endurance race. C may be true but the passage does not claim to extend the correlation to other sports so it is not a flaw. D is never stated as no other sports are mentioned. Whilst if true, E would fail to support the findings of the research mentioned in the passage it is not a flaw in that research that has been undertaken.

Question 5: D

The top 3 scores on either attempt were no. 4 1st attempt – 7.34m, no. 13 2nd attempt 7.29m, the 3rd would be no. 4's 2nd attempt (7.26m) but they have already qualified so then next best is no. 10 1st 7.17m.

Anyone else within 50cm of third place 7.17m or 717cm qualifies, so anything above (717-50 = 667cm) 6.67m qualifies

Competitor Number	1st	2nd
1		
2	✓	
3		✓
4	Already qualified	
5		✓
6		
7	✓	
8		
9		
10	Already qualified	
11		
12		
13	Already qualified	

14		✓
15		

Which totals 5 competitors in addition to the top 3 , so 5 + 3 = 8, answer D.

Question 6: C

The passage is about the impending difficulties facing African and Asian agriculture due to future climate changes that will result in food shortages. It concludes that the development of seed banks with detailed catalogues about their trait so that farmers may be able to trial crops for the future, which is expressed in C.

A and E the basis for the problem, rather than conclusions and so are wrong. B is the hopeful outcome but not the conclusion, also the closing sentence states that seed banks are not the only answer, which B implies so it is incorrect. The main conclusion is about creating seed banks, which would then allow for D, so it is more of a secondary conclusion or suggestion rather than the main conclusion.

Question 7: C

Laying out share price for each day in a table:

Monday	Tuesday	Wednesday	Thursday	Friday
£1	£1.20	x	1.25x	£1

As Wednesday's price is unknown, use x. Thursday is 125% of x.
For Helen's shares:

Monday	Tuesday	Wednesday	Thursday	Friday
£1000	£1200	x	£1350	

This means on Tuesday the shares must have been worth £1200.
$1.25x = £1350$ so $x = £1080$ *(1350 ÷ 5 x 4 = 1080)*

Monday	Tuesday	Wednesday	Thursday	Friday
£1000	£1200	£1080	£1350	

Therefore, the price change between Tuesday and Wednesday is a decrease of 10% (1200 x 0.9 = 1080).
So for Paul: £3600 x 0.9 = £2700

Monday	Tuesday	Wednesday	Thursday	Friday
	£3600	£2700		

He therefore made a loss of £300.

Question 8: B

In a direct comparison, with non-custodial sentences the rate of reoffending was 22%, for custodial sentences it was 55%, this shows that the rate of reoffending was significantly lower for those with non-custodial sentences therefore which means that it would be a mistake, as stated in B, to give a custodial sentence when a non-custodial sentence is also appropriate as doing so would likely result in a higher chance or reoffending.

A cannot be reliably concluded as we have no specific data about serving half sentences.

That " 70% of under 18s re-offend" would suggest that there are significant problems but it does not fully support C that it is a mistake to send them to prison, we would need data comparing with those given a non-custodial sentence. C is incorrect as study 1 shows that only 72% reoffend, after 9 years. Whilst they all may do eventually we have not been given the data to show this so it cannot be reliable concluded. For E we have no data on comparing rates of reoffending for short (less than 12 months) with over 12 months so again it cannot be reliably concluded.

Question 9: D
Of the 50 000 former prisoners:
➢ In year 1 44% reoffended = 22 000
➢ In year 5 66% had reoffended which is 33,000 (a further 11,000).

Question 10: A
The phrase "instead of" implies there is the choice of whether to give a community service rather than prison sentence as they are eligible for both, which would account for the limited population where this was possible, where it reduces reoffending rates by 6%. The comparison of 55% versus 22% is simply a comparison of reoffending rates for all non-custodial versus custodial sentences but it may be that many of those given a custodial sentence were not eligible for a non-custodial so a direct comparison with the group where both were available cannot be made.

Question 11: E
E if true would strengthen the argument the most as it gives evidence compared with a control group that restorative justice is 20% more effective at reducing reoffending rates than just a community service order. This provides strong evidence that restorative evidence is effective and so would strengthen the argument that more offenders should be subjected to restorative justice to reduce reoffending rates.

A would not strengthen the argument as much as it does not provide evidence for the effects of restorative justice without a prison sentence, so there is no basis for comparison for the effects on reoffending rates.

B and C are moral and practical arguments for the argument of sending to prison rather than restorative not against, so weaken the argument. D is a financial argument rather than being based on the evidence of the report.

Question 12: D

Using the possible points of 9, 5, 3 and -2, it's possible to make:

> Crosswords: $9 + 5 + 5 + 3 = 22$
> Jigsaws: $9 + 9 + 5 - 2 = 21$
> Rubiks: $9 + 9 + 3 + 3 = 2$
> Tangrams: $9 + 9 + 9 - 2 = 25$

But it is not possible to make a score of 23 so the Solitaires score must have been wrongly calculated.

Question 13: D

The argument is essentially a discussion comparing the benefits to an individual compared with the risks to society but eventually arguing that the risk of a negative message to society is not worth the risk of allowing a previously convicted criminal to return to a high profile job, this makes the assumption that the rights of the individual are less important than the risks to society, which is stated in D.

Question 14: B

For the red paint, 20ml is left so 80 ml must be used. 20% is used as red, for 10% each purple and orange half each mix is red, so a further 5% each, so 10% total. For brown red is 1/3 of the 30%, so 10%. This means 20% + 10% + 10% = 40% of the mural is red from 80ml of paint, which means each 1% is 2ml.

For blue paint 10% is blue alone, for brown the blue makes up 1/3 of 30%, = 10%, and for 10% each green and purple half of each mix is blue, so a further 5% each, so 10% each. This totals 10% + 10% +10% = 30%, and each 1% is 2ml the blue paint used is (2ml x 30% =) 60ml. So 40 ml of the 100ml of blue paint is not used.

Question 15: A

The passage explains how human and primate brains are very similar such that we should consider research on primates to understand the effects of brain lesions may help to develop treatments, this is the conclusion, A.

B, C and D are not mentioned in the passage. E would be too strong a conclusion based on the conditional tone of the passage that research 'may' help.

Question 16: D

Including Maisy there are 16 girls, and 10 boys, 26 children total.

There are no more than two children in each family.

So the 3 older girls which have younger sisters = 6 girls.

The 2 girls with brothers (and vice versa)= 2 girls and 2 boys.

The two boys with brothers = 4 boys

Which totals 8 girls and 6 boys with brothers and sisters, i.e. 14 children, so there are 12 of the 26 children without siblings.

Question 17: A

The argument states that the development of a new blood test will help reduce the rate of recorded heart attacks in women. It states that this will be because more sensitive detection will allow for earlier treatment. However it fails to take account for the fact that with more sensitive detection, the recorded rates of heart attacks in women is likely to increase, as those not previously picked up may now be, as stated in A.

Question 18: E
For the 720 points, the span goals make up 42 x 8 = 336, and beat 36 x 5 = 180, which together total 516. This leaves 720 – 516 points for tip goals, = 204 points total. This means that 102 tips were scored (as each tip scores 2)
This means that the points for span goals were roughly half, and beat and tip quarters with beat slightly smaller which is best represented in E.

Question 19: C
2 litres of sugary drink is 2000ml. 330ml contains 35g of sugar or 9 lumps. There is about 6 lots of 330ml in 2000ml. 6 x 9 lumps = 54 lumps

Question 20: C
Taking 100% of the daily-recommended sugar intake to be for example 100g. "Teenagers consume 50% more sugar on average, so 150% would be 150g. The information states that 30% is comprised of sugary drinks, which would be 30% of 150g = 45g. If this were to reduce to 1/3 as much, this would reduce by about 30g to 15g and so go from 150g to 120g, which would be the equivalent of 120% of the daily-recommended sugar, or 20% above the recommended level.

Question 21: C
If the tax resulted in a 10% reduction the 5 727 million litres of sugary drinks would reduce to about 5154 million (5727 x 0.9).

Question 22: A
If A were true it would most weaken the argument for a sales tax rather than volume tax on sugary drinks. If retailers reduced prices to remain competitive this would negate the effects of a sales tax in the attempt to reduce consumption. The increase in price with the sales tax would be counteracted by the reduction in price by the retailers to remain competitive. This would not have the same effect with a volume tax as more expensive drinks would not be as heavily taxed so there would not be the same need to reduce price by the retailers. Statements C, D and E make no comparison of the advantage of the volume versus sales tax. B only states that most food is taxed by volume but does not give any arguments for or against this rather than taxing by price.

Question 23: E
As the tourist took the shortest route, it is logical that the attraction he did not visit would be either the Tower or the Palace as these are the furthest distance from all of the others. The shortest possible route is from the hotel to the courts 60m so this will definitely be taken so it makes sense to start with this. Logically the next step is to go towards the fountain as otherwise the tourist will get to the Palace and then need to

either go to the Tower, which cannot be right as one of the Tower or Palace must be missed, or back to the hotel which would add unnecessary distance.

So he goes to the fountain 80m, then the Arch 80, the Castle 90m and then Tower 110m and finally back to the hotel 110m. This totals 530m, so the Palace is the attraction that is missed as it is not possible to do the other option of missing the Tower and doing the other 5 attractions in a 530m route.

Question 24: B

The argument states that the banning of caffeine drinks may backfire on schools exam results due to the positive effects of caffeine on focus and short-term memory. However, if statements 1 and 3 were true it would weaken the argument as they suggest that caffeine that would have negative effects on sleep, which would result in lack of focus and memory. Hence the negative effects of sleep deprivation would counteract the positive effects of caffeine itself on focus.

Question 25: F

Represent the six letters as: A-8-B-X-Y-Z.

We know that:

A8B	**and**	A8
+ XYZ		+ BX
8 0 0		+ YZ
		8 0

For the three digit sums B + Z must = 10 due to the 0 digit below, the possibilities are 7 & 3 or 6 & 4 as 8 is already taken (and Y = 1 as the second column must also sum to 0 and it will have a 1 carried).

A and X must be 5 and 2 in either order as they must sum to 8 with the carried 1. They cannot be 4 and 3 as B & Z must contain exactly one of the numbers 4 & 3 therefore making the pair incompatible. So 8 + X + Z must sum to a number with 0 as the second digit (which cannot be 10 as the only way would be 8 + 1 + 1 which would use 1 twice and therefore not be allowed). Thus, it must be 20 which gives:

$$X + Z + 8 = 20$$
$$X + Z = 12$$

From earlier we know that Z the possibilities were 7, 3, 6 or 4 and for X: 5 or 2. The only combination of these that sums to 12 is 7 and 5, so we now know that X = 5 and Z = 7. Which means that B = 3 and A = 2. So the full pass code is: 2-8-3-5-1-7

Question 26: C

The argument states that previous bad press surrounding saturated fats may have been based on misleading, now discredited data. The passage only discusses these particular studies but does not make any account for other studies that may have supported their results with more substantiated research, which is the assumption of the argument.

Question 27: C

As fewer than 5% owned neither device the total population that may overlap is about 95%. Plotting the potential overlap using the minimal overlap:

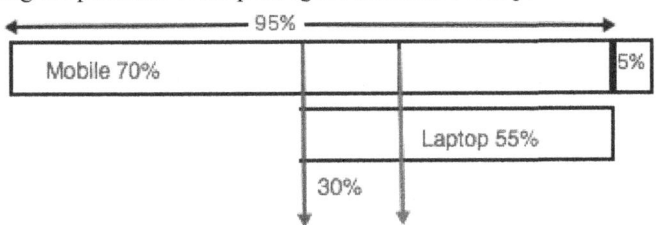

In which case the minimum overlap is 30% (70% + 50% -95%). It may be more than this if more of the mobile owners also own laptops but this is the lower bound assuming the highest potential number of children only own one device. However because the percentage that owned neither is actually **fewer** than 5%, but by how much we do not know, the potential overlap is less than 30% as the laptop owners may move further into the 5% block and so the most correct answer from the options available is 25%.

Plotting the maximum overlap:

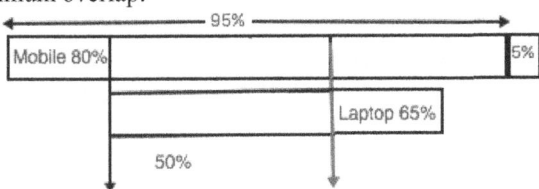

For which the overlap is 50% (80% + 65% - 95%). So, between 25 - 50%.

Question 28: A

The argument states that people are different in whether they are more alert at night or in the morning according to levels of melatonin. Consequently employers should adjust working hours to accommodate these sleeping patterns. If it were true however, that ritualistic behaviour of for example staying awake at night increases melatonin levels, this would weaken the argument, as it would suggest that the behaviour controls the melatonin levels rather than vice versa.

Question 29: A

Plotting the room:
The two larger walls are 5m x 2.5m = 12.5m², so for both walls 25m²

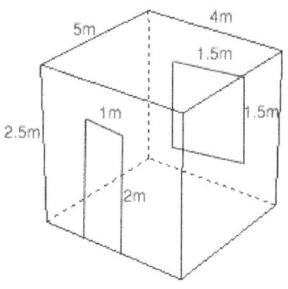

For these walls the high quality paint would need to cover 50m² and the low quality 75m².
For high quality this would need 4 tins as each covers 15m², which would cost £60 (4 x £15). For low quality this would need 5 tins, which would cost £55 (5 x £11) so for the larger walls the low quality paint is cheaper at £55.

The two smaller walls are 4m x 2.5m = 10m², so for both walls 20m². The door is 2m² and the window 3m² so with subtracting these only 15m² needs to be covered. For these walls the high quality paint would need to cover 30m² and the low quality 45m². For high quality this would need 2 tins, which would cost £30 (2 x £15). For low quality this would need 3 tins which would cost £33 (3 x £11) so for the larger walls the high quality paint is cheaper at £ 30. Therefore the total cost for the paint is £55 + £30 = £85.

Question 30: C

The argument states that because working in A&E is not attractive to doctors they will choose to work in other areas and so hospitals have to pay large sums of money for temporary staff. Which is concludes then would be to pay higher wages to the A&E doctors to provide incentive to work there which would cost the same as paying the extra temporary staff and so would be of no more net cost to the health service. If it were true that many doctors work for agencies in A&E to supplement their salaries this would strengthen the argument as it implies that doctors are incentivised by money to work in A&E and so would follow that if the wages were higher for working there more doctors would be happy to do so.

Question 31: B

From the information we know that 5 must be opposite the 6. This leaves either 2 or 1 opposite the 4 and 3.

This gives the potential combinations of the opposite sides and their totals:

> 4:2 = 6
> 4:1 = 5
> 3:2 = 5
> 3:1 = 4

Which shows that it must be 4:2 and 3:1 as the other options sum to the same totals.
Which give the pairs 5:6 = 11, 4:2 = 6, 3:1 = 4.

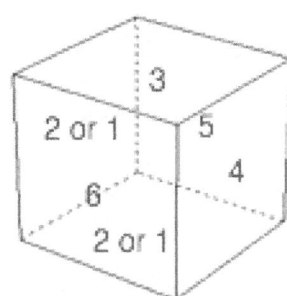 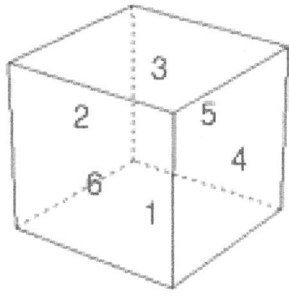

Looking at the potential answer combinations for the other die:

> A - 2:1 = 3, 3:6 = 9, so 5:4 = 9- not possible as two opposite sides would sum to 9.
> C – 4:1 = 5, 2:6 = 8, so 5:3- not possible as two opposite sides would sum to 8.
> D – 4:1 = 5, 3:6 = 9, so 2:5 = 7, not possible as 7 cannot be a total.
> E – 5:1 = 6, 2:6 = 8, so 3:4 = 7, not possible as 7 cannot be a total.
> F – 5:1 = 6, 3:6 = 9, so 2:4 = 6, not possible as two opposite sides would sum to 6.
> G – 5:1 = 6, 4:6 = 10, so 2:3 = 5 not possible as the first die has 6 as one of its totals.
> B – 2:1 = 3, 4:6 = 10, so 3:5 = 8- this is the answer as it has all different totals to itself and to the opposite die.

Question 32: G

Statement 1: from 2011-2013, 4265 defendants were convicted. But each year had about a 98% success rate of prosecution so about another 2% a year were tried and subsequently cleared. The additional 6% of 4265 is about 255 which added together is more than 430 so this is true.

Statement 2: in 2012 98% or 1552 were convicted, 1% = (1552 / 98= 15 remainder 82, so nearly 16) which means that the 2.1% acquitted was nearly 32, but definitely over 31, so this is true.

Statement 3: The total sentences handed out for includes all the suspended (220 + 178 + 140 = 538) plus the prison sentences (88 + 86 + 74 = 248). As 248 is less than half of 538, the prison sentences are represent less than 1/3 of the total sentences, so the suspended sentences represent over 2/3 so statement 3 is also correct.

All three statements are correct.

Question 33: B

If the north of England had not risen by 6.6% to 566, the number of people convicted would have been (94% of 566 =) 532. If this had, along with the rest of the country fallen by 11.7%, it would have decreased to (88% of 532 =) 469, which would have been 97 fewer convictions. $1371 - 97 = 1274$.

Question 34: C

Statement 1: is not supported as the passage only mentions how many convictions there were in West Yorkshire for 2013, not for 2012. Even for 2013 it does not say whether this was the highest increase for any region for this year.

Statement 2: is not supported as although it states that the North of England rose by 6.6% between 2012 and 2013 this is for the North of England as a whole not just for West Yorkshire, so it is not possible to confidently say that this was definitely the increase for West Yorkshire specifically, as other areas in the North may have changed by more or less and this is an average for the area.

Statement 3 is supported as in 2013 there were 1371 convictions, 566 of which were in the North which is over $\frac{2}{5}$. So, only statement 3 is supported.

Question 35: B

The argument presented in the readers comment is that rather than the North of England being particularly bad for cruelty they simply report it more as they are concerned about animal welfare. If it were true that a higher proportion of complaints resulted in conviction in the north than other regions, B, this would weaken the argument. This is because a higher conviction to complaint ratio would imply that there was not simply a higher proportion of complaints, as the reader would argue, but genuinely a higher rate of animal cruelty in the north. All of the other options do not directly address the reader's argument that the rate or reporting is higher rather than the acts of cruelty.

END OF SECTION

Section 2

Question 1: E

The reflex arc after placing a hand on a hot object

➢ Sensory neuron transmits impulse to the CNS – A
➢ Relay neuron pass electrical impulse from sensory to motor neurons – D
➢ Motor neuron transmits electrical impulse to muscle cells – C
➢ Muscle cell contracts – B
➢ So E is not part of the reflex.

Question 2: C

Alkenes will decolorise bromine water due to the presence of the C=C bond makes them unsaturated.

	Formula	Structure
1	C_2H_4	$H_2C =\!=\!= CH_2$
2	Polypropene is a polymer and has the repeating structure of $(C_3H_6)_n$	H H H H with CH₃ below each
3	$CH_2C(CH_3)_2$	$H_2C =\!=\!=$ with CH₃ and CH₃
4	CH_3CH_2I	$H_3C — CH_2 — I$

So only 3 and 1 have C=C double bond so only they will decolourise the bromine water hence C is the answer

Question 3: B

Dark, matt surfaces are better at absorbing radiation than white surfaces so black will be the better emitter of radiation. Black surfaces are also better at emitting radiation than white surfaces.

White, shiny surfaces are better reflectors of radiation so they will be better clothes in winter as they will reflect the radiation back into the person on the inside to keep them warm, and radiate the heat away less on the outside. This is true because in winter the ambient temperature is likely to be lower than the body temperature, hence the answer is B.

Question 4: B

There are 3 black beads and the total number of beads in the bag is 8.

➢ The odds of picking a black bead the first time is $\frac{3}{8}$.

➢ Having picked this the odds of picking another black bead is $\frac{2}{7}$ (the total being one less as the previous bead has been removed).

➢ To find the probability of picking two black beads multiply these odds:
$$\frac{3}{8} x \frac{2}{7} = \frac{6}{56} = \frac{3}{28}$$

Question 5: A

Anaerobic respiration is: Glucose $\Rightarrow$ lactic acid (+ little energy)

So there is no formation of carbon dioxide, use of oxygen or water formed, hence the answer is A.

Question 6: A

The energy change for the forward reaction is **a** as this is the overall energy change from reactants to products, hence the reverse reaction is **–a,** hence the answer is A.

Question 7: D

As the question says, a step down transformer decreases the voltage of an alternating current (a.c.) electricity supply. Decreasing the voltage does not decrease the power, so it **stays the same**. But as the voltage goes **down**, the current goes **up**, hence the answer is D.

Question 8: E

Drawing the triangle PQR:

To work out the tangent of angle PQR we must first workout the length of the line joining P to the midpoint of QR (M).

Using Pythagoras:

➢ $$a^2 + b^2 = C^2$$
➢ $$QM^2 + PM^2 = PQ^2$$
➢ $$4^2 + PM^2 = 6^2$$
➢ $$PM^2 = 6^2 - 4^2$$
➢ $$PM^2 = 36{-}16$$
➢ $$PM^2 = 20$$
➢ $$PM = \sqrt{20}$$

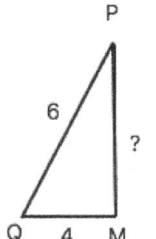

SECTION TWO

Using $Tangent = \dfrac{Opposite}{Adjacent}$

$Hence, \dfrac{\sqrt{20}}{4} = \dfrac{\sqrt{5x4}}{4}$

$Hence, \dfrac{\sqrt{5}\sqrt{4}}{4} = \dfrac{2\sqrt{5}}{4}$

$= \dfrac{\sqrt{5}}{2}$

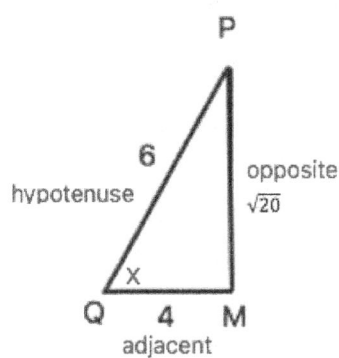

Question 9: D

The white mouse must be recessive, hence genotype cc.
The possibilities for the black mouse, 1 are CC or Cc
Punnet squares for both possibilities:

		Black	
		C	C
White	c	Cc	Cc
	c	Cc	Cc

Genotype 100% Cc + Phenotype 100% black

		Black	
		C	c
White	c	Cc	cc
	c	Cc	cc

Genotype 50% Cc, 50% cc + Phenotype 50% black, 50% white
As all of our first generation offspring are black we know that the black mouse 1, is genotype CC, and mouse 2 is genotype Cc.
A cross of these mice:

		Mouse 1	
		C	C
Mouse 2	C	CC	CC

Mouse 2			
	c	Cc	Cc

Genotype 50% CC, 50% Cc + Phenotype 100% black.

Hence 50% heterozygous (CC), black only offspring and heterozygous and homozygous genotype, hence the answer is D.

Question 10: D

Rubidium is an alkali metal and in group 1, knowing the physical and chemical properties of group 1 we know that the group 1 metals become more reactive as you move down the group, therefore is it logical to assume that being far down the group, rubidium is very reactive and would need to be stored under oil, D.

A. Is not correct as rubidium is more reactive than hydrogen and so electrolysis of rubidium chloride produces hydrogen not rubidium.

B. Is not correct as knowing the group 1 trends that melting and boiling points decrease moving down the group and so rubidium **does not** have a higher melting or boiling point than sodium.

C. Again, knowing the group 1 trends we know that rubidium reacts vigorously with water, increasing in reactivity down the group with rubidium being lower than sodium, so it is incorrect that rubidium reacts more slowly with water than sodium.

E. The chemical formula for rubidium sulphate is Rb_2SO_4, not $RbSO_4$ so this is incorrect.

Question 11: A

Statement 1 is correct – that neutrons emitted in nuclear fission can cause further fission

Statement 2 states "*the half life of a radioactive substance is half the time taken for all its nuclei to decay*", which is incorrect. The half-life of a substance is actually **the time taken for the number of radioactive isotope in a sample to halve**, which is slightly different

Question 12: B

As X is a whole number greater than zero, and most of the options are true for all values of X we can take X to be 1. Hence:

$$a = \frac{3}{5+1} = \frac{3}{6} = \frac{1}{2}$$

$$b = \frac{3+1}{5} = \frac{4}{5}$$

$$c = \frac{3+1}{5+1} = \frac{4}{6} = \frac{2}{3}$$

$$so \; a < c < b$$

To check that G is not correct try with another value, $X = 2$

$$a = \frac{3}{5+2} = \frac{3}{7}$$

$$b = \frac{3+2}{5} = \frac{5}{5} = 1$$

$$c = \frac{3+2}{5+2} = \frac{5}{7}$$

Where still $a < c < b$, hence B is correct

Question 13: B

On a hot day, a human would sweat more and lose more water, thereby making the blood plasma more concentrated. This would mean than more water is reabsorbed into the blood and the urine becomes more concentrated so there would be **less** water in the urine on a hot day compared with a cold day. Whilst the concentration of urea in urine would be affected by the volume of water, the mass of the urea will be unaffected by external temperature so the mass of urea in urine will be the **same** on a hot day compared with a cold day.

Question 14: C

Cycloalkanes are examples of alkanes, which only have single bonds, which means they are saturated, hence C is correct.

A. is incorrect as they have the general formula C_nH_{2n}
B. they do not rapidly react with bromine water. Alkenes with double C=C bonds react to decolourise bromine water
D. they burn in excess oxygen to produce carbon dioxide and water, not hydrogen, so this is incorrect
E. incorrect as they are part of a homologous series as they have similar properties and the same general formula
F. cycloalkanes are not giant covalent structures.

Question 15: A

The vertical force upwards can be deduced by subtracting the downwards force 20N from the lift from the wings 25N, (25N – 20N =) 5N.
Using the equation *force* = *mass x acceleration* and given mass = 2kg:
$5N = 2kg \, x \, a$

$$Thus \, a = 2.5ms^{-2} upwards$$

The horizontal acceleration can be deduced by subtracting the air resistance (drag) force 40N from the force from the engine 50N, (50N – 40N =) 10N.
$10N = 2kg \, x \, a$
$$Thus \, a = 5m/s^{-2} to \, the \, right$$

Question 16: E

➢ $A : B : C$
➢ 1: $\dfrac{2}{3} : \dfrac{4}{5}$
➢ $C = £3000$, which $= \dfrac{4}{5}$ so divide 3000 by 4 and multiply by 5 to find:
➢ 1, = £3750, which = A.
➢ $B = \dfrac{2}{3}$, so $\dfrac{2}{3}$ of 3750 = 2500,

Total amount collected by charity $= A + B + C$

$$= £3750 + £3000 + £2500 = £9250$$

Question 17: H

Process 1 is photosynthesis, which involves neither respiratory nor digestive enzymes. Process 2 is when the plants are eaten by the animals. Process 3 is when the carbon in animals is taken in by decomposers such as microorganisms by feeding, so both 2 and 3 involve digestive enzymes. Process 4 is when the decomposers respire, releasing the carbon as carbon dioxide to the atmosphere and so uses respiratory enzymes.

Question 18: C

The equation shown is an exothermic reaction, as shown by the negative enthalpy change. This means there is a rise in temperature as the reactions transfer energy to the surroundings. Adding a catalyst would increase not decrease the rate of reaction so A is incorrect. The state if chemical 'T' being a gas means the rate of reaction would be faster because, the surface area is increased, more particles are exposed to the other reactant, there is a greater chance of particle collision and there is greater chance of the particles colliding. Hence B is incorrect.

Increasing the temperature will increase the rate of reaction because at a higher temperature the reactant particles will have more energy and move more quickly and so collide more and more collisions result in reaction, so D is incorrect. E is incorrect because the volume of gas may not change, as all the products and reactants are gases, so there may just be a change in what the gases are rather than the volume.

The activation energy is the energy required to start the reaction, the higher the activation energy the slower the rate of reaction. This is because a high activation energy will mean that only a few particles will have enough energy to collide so the reaction will be slow, hence C is correct.

Question 19: G

V and Y represent mass numbers, which is the number of protons plus neutrons. W and X are atomic numbers, which is the number of protons.

Beta emission involves changes to the nucleus whereby a neutron is converted to a proton. This means from M to N the proton number will increase by 1, so $W + 1 = X$.

During alpha emission from N to Q the nucleus loses two protons and two neutrons, this means the mass number decreases by 4 and the atomic number decreases by 2. This means that Y will decrease by 4 when N decays to Q so $Y = V-4$.

Question 20: D

➤ m = mean
➤ n = number of pupils
➤ therefore the total score = mn

The expression for the number of pupils when another pupil is added is $n + 1$ and the mean is $m - 2$. The extra pupil scores n, so now the total score is $mn + n$.

Hence the expression for when the extra pupil takes the test and scores n:

$$\frac{mn + n}{n + 1} = m - 2$$
$$mn + n = (m - 2)(n + 1)$$
$$mn + n = mn + m - 2n - 2$$
$$n = m - 2n - 2$$
$$3n = m - 2$$
$$n = \frac{m - 2}{3}$$

Question 21: A

The question concerns the nature of aerobic bacteria and white blood cells.

1. the structure of their DNA is a double helix so this is correct
2. they both do not possess a cell wall so this is incorrect
3. they both do not possess a nucleus so this is incorrect
4. they both do possess a cell membrane so this is correct

Hence, 1 and 3 are correct.

Question 22: C

	Number of Electrons
$^{35}_{17}Cl^-$	18
$^{35}_{17}Cl^+$	16
$^{40}_{18}Ar$	18
$^{39}_{19}K^+$	18
$^{40}_{20}Ca^+$	19
$^{41}_{19}K^-$	20

The lower number is the mass number, which is the number of protons and electrons in an uncharged particle.

Thus, $^{35}_{17}Cl^-$, $^{40}_{18}Ar$ and $^{39}_{19}K^+$ all have 18 electrons in the arrangement 2.8.8 so they are the same.

Question 23: D

The reaction time is 1.4s (0.7s x 2).

The speed of the car is 20m/s

➤ *Distance = speed x time*

➤ Distance = 20 m/s x 1.4s, = 28m travelled in the reaction time.

For the braking distance the car is decelerating at a constant speed from 20 to 0 in 3.3s so can take 10 m/s for this time as this will be the average speed.

$Distance = 10 x 3.3 = 33m$

Adding the braking distance and reaction time distance: 28m + 33m = 61m

Question 24: D

$$= \frac{2x+3}{2x-3} + \frac{2x-3}{2x+3} - 2$$

$$= \frac{(2x+3)(2x+3)}{(2x-3)(2x+3)} + \frac{(2x-3)(2x-3)}{(2x-3)(2x+3)} - \frac{2(2x-3)(2x+3)}{(2x-3)(2x+3)}$$

$$= \frac{4x^2 + 6x + 6x + 9 + 4x^2 - 6x - 6x + 9 - 2(4x^2 + 6x - 6x - 9)}{(2x-3)(2x+3)}$$

$$= \frac{4x^2 + 6x + 6x + 9 + 4x^2 - 6x - 6x + 9 - 8x^2 - 12x + 12x + 18}{(2x-3)(2x+3)}$$

$$= \frac{9 + 9 + 18}{(2x-3)(2x+3)}$$

$$= \frac{36}{(2x-3)(2x+3)}$$

Question 25: G

Looking at the columns of chromosomes:

XAA = X:A 1:2 (or 0.5:1) so XAA is male, which makes answers A, B, C and D incorrect.

XYAA , the Y is irrelevant to the sex of the fruit fly so the ratio of X:A is again 1:2, or 0.5:1, so XYAA is also male, which makes answers, E and F incorrect.

At this point we are left with answers G and H, for which notably XXAA and XYAA are given as the same sex so to save time it would be wise to skip to the final column, XXYYAA.

XXAA has ratio of X: A, 1:1, so it is female

XXYAA has ratio of X:A , 1:1 so it is female.

XXYYAA has ratio of X:A, 2:2, 1:1 so it is also female, so H is incorrect, G is the correct row.

SECTION TWO

Question 26: B

To work out the excess of oxygen first work out the moles of CH_4 and CO_2.

$$Moles = \frac{Mass}{MolecularMass}$$

Molecular Mass of:

> $CH_4 = 12 + (4 \times 1) = 16$

> $CO_2 = 12 + (16 \times 2) = 44$

> $O_2 = 32$

Moles of CH_4 $= \dfrac{1.6}{16} = 0.1$

Moles of CO_2 $= \dfrac{4.4}{44} = 0.1$

So we know that the number of moles of CH_4 to make CO_2 is 0.1.

The ratio of O_2 to CH_4/CO_2 is 2:1, so therefore we must have twice as much oxygen as CH_4/CO_2.

$0.1 \times 2 = 0.2$ so there are 0.2 moles of O_2.

$Mass = MolecularMass x Moles$

$0.2 x 32 = 6.4g$

So the mass of O_2 used is 6.4g which means 1.6g of the 8g is left unreacted.

Question 27: D

Considering each statement in turn:

1. *force = mass x acceleration*
    $5.0N = 4.0$ kg x $1.25ms^{-2}$
2. *speed = wavelength x frequency*
    5.0 ms^{-1} = 1.25m x 4.0 Hz
3. *voltage = current x resistance*
    4.0 V = 1.25A x 5.0 Ω

So 1 and 2 are true.

END OF SECTION

SECTION THREE

Section 3

"Computers are useless. They can only give you answers." (Pablo Picasso)

➢ In the statement, Picasso argues that computers are useless because they are only able to supply answers of questions posed to them. A calculator, as an example of a computer is entirely useless until one enters a sum for it to solve, but it requires the human input to perform any sort of function.

➢ As an artist Picasso must have thought computers to be against his industry of creativity and indeed at the time they would have been able to contribute very little to the arts. He may have been making a wider statement about the evolution of creativity that it will never be possible for mechanical devices to be truly creative- a thought still held by many.

➢ This argument however, whilst debatable in its truth at the time when Picasso made it, is almost impossible to defend today. Computers in their many forms are almost essential to modern day life in the western world. Most people in developed countries own mobile phones, along with the plethora of computer devices; laptops, tablets, even some cars have computers.

➢ We rely on computers for a huge number of daily functions that those who lived before them could not have anticipated. From maintaining contact with people across the world to simply arranging meetings, from organising our online banking to ordering clothes and food on websites we use computers in almost every aspect of modern life.

➢ Even in medicine, computers are often used to store patient notes and be used to keep track of lab results and as a viewing platform for medical scans. Even stripped down to the bare essentials of search engines providing answers to questions, as Picasso would argue, they are still useful to us in many areas. From searching locations, to medicine where the new recommendations for treating conditions can be found via computers.

➢ The real limits of technology are changing all the time. The evolution of technology has developed from simple calculator arithmetic functions, to now virtual realities and artificial intelligence that rivals our human abilities. Computers are on the brink of being used to drive cars more safely than humans, and be able to design and create in the way that Picasso would have never thought possible. It is possible now to interact with robots in a way that could change the way we function in the future, with computers even becoming more efficient than humans in many jobs, industrial labour for example.

➢ There are still limitations of technology, in the medical world, computers cannot replace doctors as yet. The human ability to be able to look at another human and assess how unwell they may be is a long way off being mechanised. Searching flu symptoms into an online search engine, a brain tumour appears as one of the diagnoses. It takes a person to ask the right questions, even if computers may be able to help with the answers.

➢ In conclusion, Picasso's argument may have been relevant to him and his contemporaries the context of the era and abilities of computers at the time. However, it would have been difficult for him to anticipate the exponential increase in abilities of the at the time primitive computers to now almost essential devices in every day life.

"That which can be asserted without evidence, can be dismissed without evidence."(Christopher Hitchens)

➤ Hitchens means that things that are said to be true but have no physical evidence, can be dismissed as they cannot be proven. He probably is referring to religion, the proof of the existence of which has no material evidence that can be replicated and documented in a scientific fashion. In the world of science, for example, something wouldn't be simply accepted because of folklore and people believing it to be true. The very heart of the Christian religion, the existence of God for example has not been positively proven.

➤ Arguing against this however, there are many domains where beliefs are held without material evidence. In a court of law for example a person's testimony is often held without argument. It is not often the quality of the evidence but the person who gives it that is taken into account. Why then with religion do we not believe the thousands of people, both today and historically, who we would judge to be honest caring people who deeply believe that their god exists. Especially when we will sometimes take one person at their word for deciding whether someone should be convicted or exonerated for a crime.

➤ It also brings into question what we consider to be 'evidence'. Does something have to be proven by multiple people, reportable and repeatable as with scientific research? There are many scientific principles held to be 'proven with evidence' that only have one experiment to support them. The MMR vaccine being linked to autism scandal, for example was previously supported by evidence until it was later discredited. Bloodletting was the commonplace of medicine centuries ago and was believed to have evidence supporting its efficacy, where now it seems pure madness. How many things then do we hold to be true that will later be disproven as scientific techniques evolve?

➤ Equally there are probably many things that we do not as yet have evidence for that may emerge over time. We do not yet know the full mechanism of some drugs such as paracetamol for example. Do we dismiss its worth because we cannot prove it? Hitchens' statement would argue that we should, when clearly this would be a mistake.

➤ I somewhat agree with this statement. It depends on the context to which it refers. It is potentially valid for example with new medicines. We would be wrong to accept their safety and efficacy without solid scientific evidence.

➤ However, there are also many areas of medicine that cannot be dismissed just because they don't have solid material evidence. Many personal accounts of outer body and near-death experiences where they have the option to 'move towards the light' cannot be simply dismissed because they have no physical proof. It may be that such things will never be proven, or indeed disproven in the same way that we take paracetamol to be effective simply on anecdotal evidence.

➤ Ultimately it depends on where the burden of proof lies. Is it with those who propose the hypothesis that something may be true, to then confirm their theory with evidence? Or is it for those who doubt their statement to disprove it? Hitchens would argue the former, but many issues such as widely held concepts of faith and religion are arguably the latter.

When treating an individual patient, a physician must also think of the wider society.

➤ The statement means that doctors should not only consider their patient's needs but also that of the other people within society when considering treatment. It would be ridiculous, for example, for a doctor to spend all day by a patient's bedside when that may be in their specific best interests when they have their other patients to consider as well. It also means this in wider context with respect to finite resources such as medicines, hospital resources such as radiological scans and even human tissue such as blood and organs. It is not feasible in a resource-limited system such as the NHS to prioritise the patient with no regard to the expense of other patients and wider society.

➤ It is however a doctors role to place the needs of their patients above all else. Doctors have historically prioritised patients even over the law. Helping patients addicted to drugs or alcohol for example, whilst reporting them and forcing them to change their lifestyle might be what is the best for society, doctors will often ignore these societal priorities and treat the patients regardless.

➤ Equally in a society where we have a growing population many children in foster care and waiting for adoption it is not in society's interests to treat an infertile couple with IVF where otherwise they may adopt these children and accept their infertility. But it would be against the foundations of medicine to begin to deny patients the treatment that was available and best for them to force them to accept conditions such as infertility, merely to satisfy the needs of society.

➤ There are many times where the patient's interests can conflict with those of the population. Antibiotics for example, while resistance is increasing they will become increasingly precious. It would be in society's interest to ration these for only the very unwell that won't survive without them. But this would mean that many patients suffer for longer with illnesses that could easily be treated with antibiotics that are being saved for the future society's benefit.

➤ Equally with treating people that are, or are likely to become dangerous people such as serial killers. It is clearly in society's interest to not treat these people and allow them to die, but this would be completely against the ethical principle of non-maleficence and against doctors' nature and medical training.

➤ Vaccination is another key example. Often it is actually not in the individual patient's interest to receive a vaccination, they are more likely to experience side effects from the vaccine than to acquire the infection it prevents in most cases. But it is necessary to vaccinate everyone to protect the most vulnerable members of society such as the young, elderly and immunosuppressed.

➤ In conclusion, there are times that the patient's best interests contradict that of society and doctors may have to use common sense to decide where best to spend their time and limited resources. It would for many go against the foundations of medicine to deny some patients the treatment they need to satisfy the needs of society. It may however, end up as a necessity, to ration some resources such as antibiotics for those most at need to prevent the rise of resistance making them then useless to everyone else in society.

Just because behaviour occurs amongst animals in the wild does not mean it should be allowed within domesticated populations of the same species.

➢ This statement claims that there are differences in the behaviours of domesticated animals to those living in the wild. It consequently argues that just because a certain type of behaviour exists in wild animals, that does not mean it should be automatically allowed in domesticated animals as well.

➢ It could refer to the hierarchical nature of wild animals that operate in a 'survival of the fittest' modality. It is common for animals to fight each other in the wild, for example, for simple status such as with wolves to be head of the wolf pack. This behaviour would not be acceptable in domesticated animals. It would be very difficult, for example, if every time someone attempted to walk their dog in the park it attacked other dogs to assert status, and this was allowed or even encouraged as they behaviour was fitting with its analogous species in the wild. Quite apart from the danger this might pose to the other dogs if this behaviour was encouraged, it could even lead to a change in behaviour of the fighting dog such as aggression towards humans that would make it not only impractical but dangerous to keep it as a pet.

➢ Equally with hunting where animals such as wolves and big cats would hunt their food in the wild it would be obscene to allow the domesticated versions to keep attacking other people's house bunnies or guinea pigs to satisfy their carnal nature.

➢ Arguing against the statement however, one could argue that if we are having to continually disrupt our domesticated animal's behaviour to fit with what works practically within our society, then it may be best to not keep these animals as pets. Changing the nature of these animals through behavioural modification, known as taming is arguably immoral and unfair to these animals. Training dogs to be more docile and fight their animalistic instincts on the face of it seems immoral and unfair. One could argue that just because we can force these animals to change their behaviours does not mean that we should.

➢ With breeding programmes for example, our pets have been slowly bred to be less like their historic ancestors to be more aesthetically pleasing. Whilst the taming of certain behaviours to prevent harm to other animals and even humans can be justified, it is hard to accept the alteration of animals' natural breeding behaviour for aesthetics. This has even gone to extremes where selective breeding of pugs and other dogs have been bred to their detriment as they often have breathing and other health problems.

➢ However, it is also impossible to avoid the fact that domesticated animals would ultimately not be kept as pets had their behaviour not been altered through time. So it could be argued that these changes are necessary for their existence, and so merely a form of survival adaptation. Indeed they have been so successful that they don't rival the top of the food chain humans and are even protected by them.

➢ In conclusion while modifying the behaviours of domesticated animals is ideologically difficult, it is vital to continue to allow their existence as a valued and cared for part of our society.

END OF PAPER

SECTION THREE

2016

Section 1

Question 1: D

In order to solve this question, we have to fill in the blanks in the table. Years 1 – 3 are easy as there is only one gap to fill, years 4 and 5 are a little more difficult. From the totals we can calculate the total number of boys and girls in all 5 years.

We can calculated the total number of students in year 4: 120-24-26-40-24=16

We also know that that the probability of a boy being in year 4 is 1/12, applying this we can calculate the number of bin year 4: 72/12=6.

Since we know that there are 16 students in year 4 and 6 of them are boys, the probability of a student being a boy is 6/16 or 3/8.

Year	Boys	Girls	Total
1	18	6	24
2	16	24	40
3	8	8	16
4	6	10	16
5	24	0	24
Total	72	48	120

Question 2: B

Answer A is incorrect as the forest fires in Indonesia represent only a fraction of the net allowance of CO_2 emission and there is no information on further culprits, therefore failing as a valid the conclusion.

Answer B is correct as the text specifically mentions that only CO_2 from burnt plant material is taken up by new vegetation. Due to the fact, that there is also peat being burnt in the forest fires allows the conclusion that some of the CO_2 will not be taken up by regrowth.

Answer C is incorrect as it has no backing from the text presented in the question.

Answer D is incorrect, as it basically ties in with Answer A, they both ignore other contributing factors to CO_2 emission.

Question 3: B

This question is pretty straight forward. First, calculate the price per stay and compare.

Stay 1:
Hotel: $50 + $50 + $40 + $40 + $40 = $220
Car: 5 x $5 = $25
Total: $25 + $220 = $245
Stay 2:
Hotel: 8 x $40 = $320
Car: $25 + $5 = $30
Total: $350
Difference: $350 - $245 = $105

Question 4: B

Answer A is incorrect as this is a direct rephrasing of the second sentence, therefore not a flaw. Answer B is correct, as if the ability to synchronize to particularly slow music was an innate ability of musicians that occurs naturally, there's a chance that non-musicians would have the same trait, despite not having taken up music. Answer C is incorrect as it is not supported by the text and is also irrelevant. Answer D is incorrect as whilst it might generally speaking be true, the text passage here deals with synchronization to slow music, not with any other abilities.

Question 5: A

The first challenge in this question is to correctly identify the axes of the diagram.
Looking at the distribution of results, the Y axis must represent the written paper in steps of 10 and the X axis must represent the score of the practical paper in steps of 5. Both start at 0.
Moving from left to right, the dots therefore represent the following students:
Ina – Liz – Els – Joe – Fio – Gho – Amy – Kai – Ben – Den – Haz.
Con would fall between Fio and Gho.

Question 6: D

Answer A is incorrect as the new changes do not make it more difficult to seek justice per se, but only for claims of £200 000 or more.
Answer B is incorrect since fees associated with the court cases have been in place for a long time and the text only takes issue with the recent rise, not fees as a whole.
Answer C is incorrect for similar reasons as answer A. The statement is too general for a rather narrow answer.
Answer D is correct since it is in keeping with the text as a whole.
Answer E is incorrect as they address and issue beyond the scope of the text.

Question 7: D

To answer this, we need to use a two step approach. First, it is easiest to work backwards from the answers provided to determine the amount of taxes Paul would be paying for the respective incomes. We know that Paul must be paying $4800 ($5600 - $800). In addition to that, we also know that Paul makes more money this year than he did the year before, but pays less tax. This is only possible by crossing the 50 years of age boundary. For this reason, the correct answer is D rather than C, despite the net tax payment being the right amount in both cases.

Income	Tax if under 50	Tax if over 50
$24000	$3000	$2000
$29000	$4000	$3000
$33000	$4800	$3800
$38000	$6500	$4800
$43000	$7700	$5800

Question 8: C
For this question we have to look at figure 1 as well as figure 3. From Fig 1 we know that there were 800 units of products 1, 2 and 3 sold in April to June and none of product products 4, 5 and 6 since they have not been released yet.

Looking at Fig 3 we can determine the cost for each set of **100 units**:
Income from product 1 was 8x£1500=£12000
Income from product 2 was 8x£2000=£16000
Income from product 3 was 8x£1500=£12000
Total Income: £40000

Question 9: D
From the diagram in Figure 2 we know that in the 4 month that product 2 has been on sale by June, a total of 1700 units had been sold. We also know from the question that the 900 units sold in March represent 2/3 of the sales for the months of March to May. If we define X as the number of units sold from March to May, we can express this as 900 = X x 2/3, solving this for X gives X = 1350.

Therefore, the number of units of product 2 sold in June must be 1700 – 1350 = 350. We know from Figure 3 that 100 units of product 2 are worth £2000, which means that in the month of June the sale of product 2 generated £700 income (£2000 x 3.5 = £7000).

Question 10: D
From figure 1 we know that there were 600 units of product 6 sold in November and December. Using the data from figure 3 this equates to an income of 6x£4000=£24000. From Figure 2 we can see that the income produced from product 6 in December was £6000 and therefore the income from November must be £24000-£6000=£18000. This

value is equivalent to 450 units of product 6, since £18000/£6000=4.5 and since prices are given for batches of 100 units, the result is 450 units sold in November.

Question 11: E
To solve this, you will have to calculate the total number of units sold in a year and divide this by the months since release. For product 1 this is 12, product 2 it is 10, product 3 it is 8, for product 4 it is 6, for product 5 this is 4 and for product 6 this is 2.

Product	Total sale since release	Average monthly sale since release
Product 1	3000	250
Product 2	3200	320
Product 3	2600	325
Product 4	1200	200
Product 5	1400	350
Product 6	600	300

Question 12: D
When Helen goes to bed it is 21mins to 2300, meaning it is 2239. When Helen wakes up it is 23mins to 0400, meaning 0337. Therefore Helen has slept from 2239 to 0337 which means she has slept 4hrs and 48 minutes.

Question 13: A
Answer A is correct since sports and entertainment are provided as specific exemptions to high IQ professions that are well paid by the text.
Answer B is incorrect since the IQ is independent of education.
Answer C is incorrect as the statement misinterprets the argument of the text that specifically states that the research did not consider parental profession when analysing IQs.
Answer D is incorrect as it argues a point beyond the scope of the text.

Question 14: D

The easiest way to approach this question is to calculate the balance per month.

Month	Balance	Month	Balance
January	$1300	July	$1100
February	$1100	August	$1300
March	$1300	September	$1200
April	$1300	October	$1500
May	$1700	November	$1400
June	$1500	December	$1400

Sam has **over $1300** in her account in May, June, October, November and December.

Question 15: B

Answer A is incorrect since the text makes no claim about unhealthy lifestyle accelerating synapse loss in old age.

Answer B is correct since the text claims that healthy lifestyles can produce additional synapses meaning that after age related synapse loss there are a higher number of synapses still available.

Answer C is incorrect as it has nothing to do with the text.

Answer D is incorrect since the link between quality of life and existing synapses is not mentioned in the text.

Answer E is incorrect since it does not provide a relevant conclusion to the topic addressed in the text.

Question 16: A

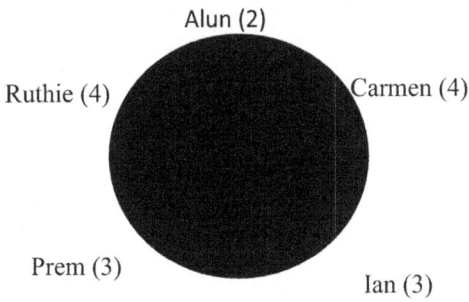

After Alun's throw, he has 0 coins, Ruthie has 7 coins and Carmen has 7 coins.
After Carmen's throw, she has 2 coins, Alun has 1 coin and Ian has 7 coins.
After Ian's throw he has 2 coins, Carmen has 4 coins and Prem has 6 coins.
After Prem's throw she has 1 coin, Ian has 3 coins and Ruthie has 9.
After Ruthie's throw he has 4 coins, Alun has 2 coins and Prem has 3 coins.

Question 17: A

Answer A is correct since only the regulation of use of these new antibiotics will maintain their effect on bacteria.

Answer B is incorrect since it neither strengthens or weakens the argument but rather provides more background information.

Answer C is incorrect since it has nothing to do with the topic discussed in the text.

Answer D is incorrect since it has little relevance for the incentive provided to pharmaceutical companies to research new antibiotics.

Question 18: D

To solve this, it is easiest to calculate the interest for the 1st year for the individual mortgages this person qualifies for.

Since he already has £25000 and wants a house worth £150000, he needs to cover approximately 83% of the house through a mortgage. This means he does not qualify for Mortgages 1 and 2.

To calculate the interest for year 1, we need to apply the respective percentages to the mortgage amount of £125000.

Mortgage No	Year 1 Interest	Arrangement Fee	Year 1 Total Cost
3	£6250	£500	£6750
4	£3750	£2000	£5750
5	£5000	£1000	£6000

Mortgage 4 is the cheapest in year 1, resulting in answer D.

Question 19: C

To calculate this, we need to calculate the growth for Texas, where the number of new wells in 2012 represents roughly 40% (40.11%) of the wells drilled in from 2005 – 2011.

40% of 2694 = 1077.6 which roughly equates to answer C.

Question 20: C
To answer this, we need to calculate the net water use per well. This is easiest using approximate numbers:
For Louisiana: 12000/2500= 4.8 million gallons per well.
For Utah: 600/1200=0.5 million gallons per well.
Difference between Louisiana and Utah: 4.8 – 0.5 = 4.3 million gallons per well. Since we used approximation we will use the next closest answer, which is C.

Question 21: E
Statement 1 is correct since the risk is specifically mentioned in the text as the last sentence in the 'Chemicals used' paragraph and according to the table Texas used 110000 million gallons of water, equating to 99.2% of the fracking fluid. Therefore, they must have used 880 million gallons of chemicals.

Statement 2 is incorrect since the total amount of pollution produced equates to 28 coal power plants per the text which means that one power plant equates to 100,551,000/28 = 3,591,107 tonnes of carbon dioxide, not 36,000,000 tonnes carbon dioxide.

Statement 3 is correct since the text states that 26 000 million gallons are enough to supply 200,000 Colorado households for a year meaning that each household uses 26,000 million/200,000 = 130 000 gallons of water.

Question 22: H
Statement 1 does not provide an explanation for the difference in water consumption per well since the amount of water required for the process is independent from the amount of water available as mentioned by the text quoting the draught in Texas.

Statement 2 does not provide an explanation as the development in technology as it does not explain the degree of variability in water consumption, even if we assume that the fundamental understanding of technological progress is to equate in a reduction of water consumption.

Statement 3 does not provide an explanation since the per well water consumption for states varies, as demonstrated by question 20.

Question 23: D

Answer A is incorrect since it ignores the square as demonstrated by the proximity of the right and down pointing diagonal to the circle.

Answer B is incorrect since the angle of what is supposed to be the larger triangle is incorrect.

Answer C is incorrect since it misrepresents the position of the circle on the different cards.

Answer D is correct.

Answer E is incorrect since it ignores the square card.

Question 24: C

Answer A is incorrect since it is irrelevant as the text has already demonstrated the effectiveness of high impact walking irrespective of age and gender.

Answer B is incorrect since it is too specific and does not account for a general weakening of the argument.

Answer C is correct since it provides a general explanation for why the weight loss effect of playing sports is less marked.

Answer D is incorrect since it is irrelevant for the argument in the text that addresses the effect on BMI rather the motivation for performing a certain type of exercise.

Question 25: D

To answer this question we have to calculate the overall time that elapses between the start of the showings at 1015 and the end of the showings at 2245 which is 12.5hrs or 750mins.

Since the time between films is the same throughout the day, we can simply add up the duration of all the showings: $2 \times (117 + 109 + 119) = 690\text{mins}$

The total amount of time spent on breaks therefore is $750 - 690 = 60\text{mins}$.

Since 2245 marks the end of the 6th showing 60mins has to be distributed over 5 equal rest intervals: $60/5 = 12\text{mins}$.

Question 26: B

Answer A is incorrect since it has no relevance for the text that addresses the effectiveness of the mentioned self-help books not the attainability of a happy life.

Answer B is correct since this is the population that would most benefit from the purchase of a self–help book about happiness.

Answer C is incorrect since this possibility is already accounted for by the text through the use of 'are more **likely** to be anxious…'.

Answer D is incorrect since it has no relevance for the text that specifically addresses the connection between self-help books and anxiety and not the lack of a connection.

Question 27: F

There are two ways to answer this question.

Firstly, you can approach this from a theoretical perspective. In order to maximize the difference between systole and diastole, we have to have a very high systolic reading or a very low diastolic reading. Therefore, you can scan the diastolic column for the lowest readings (78 and 81) and find the combination with the highest associated systolic reading. To then ensure that you have not missed anything, check your result against the highest systolic reading.

The second option is to work backwards from the solutions looking at the differences for all the days of the respective pulse number presented in the answer.

Question 28: D

Answer A is incorrect since the text specifically mentions a degree of uncertainty in the last sentence.

Answer B is incorrect since it oversimplifies the issue with regards to the information presented in the text.

Answer C is incorrect since the text is not about cancer prevention but about what brings cancer about.

Answer D is correct since only with some influence on pollution and stress can a patient take control over them developing cancer as claimed in the last sentence.

Question 29: B

In order to find the solution for this, it is easiest to follow the instructions step by step drawing them out:

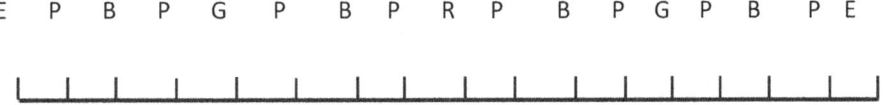

The second approach is to use the folding pattern for help. We know that the number of strands doubles on each fold, moving from 1 to 2 to 4 to 8. Since the green mark is added at the 2-strand-stage, half of the marks on the respective strands will lie between the two green marks. This means, that we will add 2 blue marks as there are 4 strings and 4 purple marks as there are 8 strands. Then, we need to add the single mark of red since it will provide the mid-point of the overall string that must necessarily lie between the two green marks.

Question 30: D

Answer A is incorrect since it is an absolute value ignoring the concept of the text itself.

Answer B is incorrect since the text does not aim to provide a time frame but merely highlight the possibility of consciousness developing in machines.

Answer C is incorrect for similar reasons as Answer A.

Answer D is correct since the connection between consciousness and brain function is unclear even when dealing with living creatures such as animals.

Question 31: D

The best way to approach this is to set up an equation.

X = points achieved by the Argents

Z = number of fesses achieved by the Sables

Y = number of fesses achieved by the Argents

X = 11Y since the Argents achieves twice as many pales as fesses and X is total number of points

X − 1 = 9Z since the Sables achieved the same number of fesses as pales

Z − 1 = Y since the Argents achieved one less fess than the Sables

Z − 1 = Y since the Argents achieve one less fess than the Sables.

Therefore Z = Y + 1.

Combining the points achieve we get 9Z + 1 = 11Y.

Insert the value of Z we have calculated above:

9Y + 10 = 11Y and solve for Y to get 5 = Y

Since Y is the number of fesses scored by the Argents, and they achieved twice as many pales as fesses, they must have scored 10 pales which is answer D.

Question 32: A

The answer from this can be found in the Table in the column giving total amount of polyunsaturated. For Olive Oil this is 10% and for Sunflower oil this is 65.7%. Since they both occur in a 50:50 mix the easiest way to find the solution is to add half of the content of each meaning 5% from the Olive Oil and 32.85% from the Sunflower Oil This leads to 37.85% which can be rounded up to 37.9%.

Question 33: A

Answer A is correct since it specifically says so in the text in the second paragraph in the last two lines.

Answer B is incorrect since the constituents of diets in hunter-gatherer societies around the world vary according to climate.

Answer C is incorrect since the third paragraph specifically mentions that the fall in heart disease is associated with the consumption of polyunsaturated fats.

Answer D is incorrect since the text specifically contradicts this by pointing out the cardio protective nature of high polyunsaturated fat oils.

Answer E is incorrect since the heart protective effect has improved with a higher ratio.

Question 34: B
According to the text the average adult ingests 143 grams of fat of which 30% are vegetable oil which equates to 43g.

Since 100g of Canola oil contain 0.6g of Erucic acid, this equates to roughly 0.26g (260mg) of Erucic acid which equates to just over 50% of the daily suggested intake.

Question 35: D
We know from the table that Sunflower oil does not contain any omega 3 so can only contribute Omega-6.

Similarly we know that the ratio of Omega-6 to Omega-3 in flaxseed oil is 0.2:1. For this is easiest to work with 100g of flaxseed oil and work out how much sunflower oil has to be added to achieve the 2:1 ratio.

Since Flaxseed oil contains 53.3g of Omega-3 we need to achieve 106.6g of Omega-6 in the mix.

12.7g of that are already contained in the flaxseed bolus, meaning we need to add the equivalent of roughly 94g of Omega-6 from sunflower oil. The amount of sunflower oil is (94/65.7)x100g = 143g.

This means the mixture of oils will weigh 243g. Looking at this we can approximate that the flaxseed oil representing slightly less than half of the mass. The closest percentage to this is 41% from answer D.

Calculation: 100/243 = 0.411 = 41%.

END OF SECTION

Section 2

Question 1: D

Answer A is incorrect since the vessels are named incorrectly.

Answer B is incorrect since the vessels are named correctly, but the content of urea is not allocated correctly.

Answer C is incorrect since the vessels are named incorrectly.

Answer D is correct since the structures are named correctly and so is the urea concentration.

Answer E is incorrect since the structures are named incorrectly.

Answer F is incorrect since the structures are named incorrectly.

Question 2: F

Statement 1 is incorrect - no element is in both period 3 and group 12.

Statement 2 is correct since the element has up to 3 electrons to donate and oxygen can take up 2 with the smallest common denominator being 6.

Statement 3 is correct since Br can take up one electron and the compound has 3 to donate.

Statement 4 is correct since elements will contain the same number of protons as they contain electrons meaning that the atomic number must be 13.

Statement 5 is incorrect since alkali metals are only in group 1.

Question 3: D

From the diagram, we know that two pieces of the material displace 100 cm³, therefore 1 piece must displace 50 cm³.

The weight difference from no pieces of material to one piece of material is 300g.

Therefore, the correct formula to use must be 300g/50cm³.

Question 4: A

First, we need to establish the slope of the line that passes through the two points given in the question using the $y = mx + b$ equation:

$$m = \frac{(y_2 - y_1)}{(x_2 - x_1)} \text{ Meaning m} = \frac{2}{3}$$

To determine b we need to insert one of the two points into the equation: $y = \frac{2}{3}X + b$:

Using $(\frac{6}{9})$ this gives $9 = \frac{2}{3}x6 + b$; solve for b to find b = 5.

Therefore the equation is $y = \frac{2}{3}X + 5$.

Since two lines are parallel if they have the same slope, the only possible answer is A where the slope (m) is 2/3.

Question 5: B

W must be a chromosome since it is the origin of the removed DNA.

X must be a restriction enzyme since it removes cuts the DNA strand to remove the DNA fragment.

Y must be a restriction enzyme since it cuts a gap into the DNA of the other organism.

Z must be a ligase since only ligase enzymes can fuse DNA strands which will result in insertion of chromosome DNA into the other organism.

Question 6: E

Answer A is correct since removing water from a solution of calcium carbonate and water will leave solid calcium carbonate.

Answer B is correct since the two substance will have different vaporisation points due to different molecular size.

Answer C is correct since silicon dioxide is a solid that poorly dissolves in water allowing filtration as an effective means of separation.

Answer D is correct since the vaporisation point of sodium chloride and water is different.

Answer E is incorrect since ethanol and water form a solution that cannot be separated by mechanical means but only by thermic separation techniques.

Question 7: D

Statement 1 is correct since the difference in weight is due to different numbers of neutrons in the core that will not change the chemical properties of the element.

Statement 2 is correct since the atomic number is due to the number of protons.

Statement 3 is incorrect since all the isotope nuclei contain 28 protons but a varying number of neutrons.

Question 8: B

The easiest way to solve this is via an equation where we assume that N consists of a number of people all weighing exactly 75kg and that Jim, Karen and Leroy each weigh 90kg.

$$78 = \frac{[75N + (3x\,90)]}{N + 3}$$

Solving this equation for N, leads to N = 12, which is solution B.

Question 9: F

From statement 1 we know that the enzyme must be in the stomach as the stomach is the only place in the human body with a pH of below 4.

From statement 2 we know that the enzyme must be a protease as it digests proteins into amino acids.

From statement 3 we know that the enzyme must be inside the body.

Answer A is incorrect as amylase digests sugars.

Answer B is incorrect as amylase digests sugar.

Answer C is incorrect as lipase digests fat.

Answer D is incorrect as lipase digests fat.

Answer E is incorrect since the pH in the small intestine is above 4.

Question 10: F

To solve this we need to count elements and add the respective molecular weight.

N = 14, there are 2 in the equation leading to 28.

H = 1, there are 20 in the equation leading to 20.

Fe = 56, there is 1 in the equation leading to 56.

S = 32, there are 2 in the equation leading to 64.

O = 16, there are 14 in the equation leading to 224.

In total this adds up to 392, which is answer F.

Question 11: B

Rotating the coil at a faster constant speed will accelerate the voltage change thereby increasing the amplitude and since the coil will also complete its turns faster, the frequency of the waves will increase as well. Only answer B ticks these boxes.

Question 12: D

This is a two part question. First we need to find the radius of the arterial lumen and then apply the equation defining the area of a circle to this.

Since the overall diameter of the artery is 1.6cm and the walls are 1mm thick, the inside diameter is 1.4cm, leaving the radius to be 7mm.

Since $A = \pi r^2$, $A = \pi \times 7^2 = 49\pi$ mm^2

Question 13: B

Carbon dioxide is only produced in aerobic respiration since it requires oxygen which per definition is absent in anaerobic respiration. Glucose represents the energy substrate in either type of respiration. Lactate is only produced in anaerobic respiration.

Question 14: C

Answer A is incorrect since the cathode would give form Hydrogen as the Calcium is more reactive.

Answer B is incorrect as the anode would give oxygen since the nitrate is a complex ion.

Answer C is correct.

Answer D is incorrect since products are allocated to the wrong electrodes.

Answer E is incorrect since molten NaCl does not contain any hydrogen.

Question 15: D

Firstly, all waves named in the question travel at the speed of light which is defined as 3×10^8 m/s or 300 000 km/s.

Since the distance from satellite to transmitter and receiver is 45,000 km each, the waves must travel 90 000 km, which will take $= \dfrac{90,000}{300,000} = 0.3s$

Secondly, we know from the question that the waves have a frequency of 1.5×10^{10}Hz, which defines them as microwaves, which leads to answer D.

Question 16: C

To solve this question, we have to work in several steps as we need to calculate both the length of RS and the length of PQ.

To calculate RS we need to know that tan is defined as opposite/adjacent, in this case RS/6. Since the question gives us the tan as 4/3, we know that RS must be 8.

RS/6 = 4/3 = 8/6.

Appling this we can calculate the area to be $A = \left(5x8\right) + \left(\dfrac{6x8}{2}\right)$

$= 40 + 24 = 64cm^2$

Question 17: G

Statement 1 is correct, this is known as a gain of function mutation.

Statement 2 is correct, this is known as a loss of function mutation.

Statement 3 is correct, this is known as a loss of function mutation.

Statement 4 is correct, this is known as a gain of function mutation.

Question 18: E

We know from the question that the acid is able to donate two protons therefore we know that we must use twice the volume of NaOH, which is able accept 1 proton.

Since the concentration of NaOH is half of that of the diprotic acid, we need 4 times the amount of the solution provided in the question to neutralize the acid.

Since the volume of the acid is given as 30cm³, we need 120cm³ (4x30cm³) of NaOH.

Question 19: D

Since we don't know the resistance of the body, the best formula to use here to find the current is I = Coulombs/time in seconds.

First, we need to calculate the charge in Coulombs (1 Coulomb = 1 joule per volt):

$\dfrac{125J}{500V} = 0.25$ C

Therefore $I = \dfrac{0.25C}{0.01s} = 25A$

Question 20: C

The main point here is not to lose the overview over the different components of the equation. Then there is no real trick to this, other than going through it step by step:

$$\frac{a}{b} = \frac{c}{d} + \frac{e}{f}$$

$$\frac{a}{b} = \frac{fc + de}{df}$$

$$dfa = bfc + bde$$

$$dfa - bfc = bde$$

$$\frac{f(da - bc)}{da - bc} = \frac{bde}{da - bc}$$

$$f = \frac{bde}{da - bc}$$

Question 21: A

Statement 1 is correct as it basically aims at the doubling of the genetic material which happens through the process of mitosis.

Statement 2 is incorrect since growth happens through the production of proteins which does not occur during mitosis.

Statement 3 is incorrect since again this happens through protein production, which is halted during mitosis.

Statement 4 is correct since stem cell division follows the same principle as asexual reproduction.

Question 22: B

Due to the increased concentration of the acid, twice that of the original sample, the reaction speed will be higher, but as the net amount of the acid in the sample is the same as in the original experiment, half the mass at twice the concentration, the equilibrium will be the same. Only line B fits this bill.

Line A equates to higher concentration and higher net amount.

Line C equates to lower concentration of acid and the same net amount.

Line D equates to a lower net amount of acid.

Line E equates to a lower concentration as well as a lower net amount of acid.

Question 23: E

From the information given in the question we know that the object must weigh 1.5kg on earth (15N at g=10N/kg).

The mass of the object will remain unchanged as it is transported to the planet. The difference will be due to the different gravitational fields.

Since we know from the text that the object has a weight of 3N on the planet, it will have a kinetic energy of 30N after a fall of 10m.

Question 24: D

This question deliberately aims to confuse you with additional information. The population distribution of the different blood groups is not needed to answer this question. There are 4 different blood groups A, B, AB and 0. One individual can have one of those 4 blood types. Since the question asks about the probability of the one criminal having both A and B antigens, he/she must have blood group AB, the likelihood of which is 25% or ¼.

Question 25: H

From the diagram, we can deduce that a grey coat colour must be dominant and a white coat colour must be recessive. Therefore, any grey mouse can potentially be heterozygous. There are 12 grey mice in the diagram, leaving answer H.

Question 26: D

From the equation, we know that the volume of the final product will be equivalent to the volume contribution of X. Since we use 100cm³ of reagent X and the reaction occurs under exclusion of air and to completion, the final volume in the syringe must be 100cm³.

Question 27: C

The easiest way to answer this question is to calculate backwards to determine the wavelength of the light through air.

We know that 360nm equates to ¾ of the wavelength through air; if X = wavelength through air: 360nm = X x 0.75

X = 480nm.

If Y is defined as the wavelength of light through glass, we can express this as

Y = 480nm x 2/3 which gives Y = 321.6nm.

Section 3

'You can resist an invading army; you cannot resist an idea whose time has come.'
(Victor Hugo)

➢ In this question, Hugo basically evaluates the strength of physical confrontation and violence versus intellect and words when it comes to changing the status quo. This position has to be connected to be taken in connection with his time. It has to be taken into account that he lived in France just after the Revolution and during the reinstitution of the monarchy in France. You can also remove the quote completely from the historical background and look more at the conflict between forced change and passive change with the invading army representing forced change and the idea a more passive and natural form of change. The forced change does not necessarily have to come in the form of an invading army consisting of battalions of soldiers but can also represent something as simple as a prescribed mind-set or political conviction that is propagated by a political regime.

➢ Arguing against this statement, it is obvious that sufficient force seems to be able to suppress most ideas, especially if execution of opposing violence is well publicised and very large scale. One example of this would be the wide ranging suppression of individuals in dictatorships such as North Korea where dissidence is not only punished physically but also enforced by a high degree of isolation. In the end, if it is possible to enforce a perception that any form of dissent will result in personal injury and in the injury of loved ones, violence can suppress ideology, especially if punishment is highly excessive.

➢ A further point to consider when arguing against the statement in the question is the definition of "idea whose time has come". Considering the vagueness of this point, it provides a good target for arguing against the statement as it renders the statement as a whole rather moot.

➢ The idea of physical and psychological violence versus ideas is also discussed in other works of literature such as 1984, some of the means by which though control can be achieved in the book provide good examples to add to an essay.

➢ Addressing the point of the power of ideas, there are many examples in history than can be used for this. The American Revolution presents one of them, so does the resistance against Nazi occupation in France or other countries during the Second World War In all cases ideology refused to be intimidated by violence. In this context however it is essential to highlight that ideas usually achieve power by encouraging to violence thereby almost resulting in a circular argument. The probably most obvious exception to this rule is Ghandi's peaceful disobedience promoting Indian independence without use of violence.

➢ In this question you can generally speaking take multiple routes, either staying rather close to historical examples or move in a more philosophical direction, looking at the issue with a broader perspective in mind. The challenge of the latter option is that it will be easier to lose track of your arguments and more difficult to maintain relevance of the points you make with regards to the original question.

➢ This is a very interesting question as it challenges the idea of progress in general to a certain extend as it attempts to quantify the influence of eternal stressors on the intellectual development of a society.

Science is not a follower of fashion nor of other social or cultural trends.

➢ The statement attempts to explain and understand the reasoning behind scientific progress and the interaction between science and culture and other influences on social progress. The basic assumption of this sentence is that science develops independent of other social driving forces that may or may not be subject to trends and temporary interests.

➢ In order to write a good essay you have to be clear for yourself what you understand by science, fashion and social/cultural trend.

  • Science in general is defined as the endeavour of searching for new information and truths in order to widen the horizon of our knowledge and out understanding of the world around us. In addition to that, science also has a certain set of rules that define the value and the truthfulness of the information that is being found.

  • Fashion as well as cultural trends both essentially go in the same direction. They both describe temporary and variable perceptions and interests within society. What is important in this is that trends as well as fashions tend to be variable from individual to individual or from group to group. This makes it different from science since science claims to hold an overarching always valid truth.

➢ The basic idea when arguing to the contrary is to provide arguments of why science is indeed influenced by fashions and trends. There are several ways this can be done. On one hand, you can argue from a sort of social perspective putting fashion and trends into context with social interests. This is a good starting point as it makes it clear how science and the areas of research that individuals are interested in are influenced by what fascinates the masses at any given point in time. One example for this is for example the great degree of progress in military technology in the early 20th century when Europe was ravaged by war and there was a great degree of militarism throughout many levels of society.

➢ On the other hand, you can argue in a different direction illustrating the relationship between science and trends by starting at scientific discovery and arguing its influence on trends and fashion. One example for this would be the progress in nuclear technology in the 1950s when society began dreaming about nuclear powered cars etc and the strive for new technology and the idea of progress through technology was very wide spread, in particular in the US.

➢ Other examples include the great social interest in geography and the natural sciences in general during the age of discovery of the Americas. The idea of widening frontiers and pushing civilization onwards became a great social driving force contributing to large amounts of funding as well as large movements of populations to these newly discovered lands. This also directly reflects social issues in the European heartland that made a new live abroad more favourable and attractive.

➢ When phrasing your agreement or disagreement, it pays to be direct with your opinion since this will make it easier to present your point in a direct and efficient fashion. However, be sure to have argued your points appropriately before voicing your opinion.

The option of taking strike action should not be available to doctors as they have a special duty of care to their patients.

➢ In general, when arguing this point you have to be aware of the implications of this question. You have to keep in mind that the essay you write will be shown to any admitting university that may or may not use your essay during the interview. For this reason, it may be wise to be a little careful with what you write in this type of essay. This applies to essays of this scope in general.

➢ Now, when t comes to arguing this particular essay, there are several bases you have to appreciate. Firstly, there is the nature of the relationship between doctors and their patients. As doctors we have a complicated relationship with our patients in the sense that we know many intimate details about our patients but at the same time we need to keep a professional distance to make the decisions that we deem in the patient's best interest. This tight bond between patients and doctors makes for a relationship between recipient and donor of a service that is not found outside the health care setting. Secondly you have to consider the purpose of strike action.

➢ Doctors going on strike is never an easy decision, particularly due to the sometimes live and death nature of health care. With doctors not working, the care that these vulnerable patients need may not be deliverable. This can be argued to be a direct violation of the basic ethical pillar of 'do no harm', since the doctor knowingly and without direct external pressure decides to withhold treatment that may alleviate the patient's suffering. The other ethical pillar that can be argued to be violated by doctors going on strike is the idea of beneficence, since it is the doctors duty to always act in the patient's best interest, which withholding of treatment most definitely is not.

➢ The most significant justifying reason for supporting doctors strikes is the fact that poor working conditions will necessarily have a direct influence on the doctors performance which in turn will have negative and detrimental effects on patient care. Good examples of this are fatigue due to long working hours or unsafe levels of staff due to general unattractiveness of the profession or widespread symptoms of exhaustion in the work force.

➤ Another point to consider is the reason why doctor strikes are an issue in the NHS and not as much in other countries and health care systems. This will give you a good chance to demonstrate that you have an understanding of how the NHS works and how health care is provided in different countries.

➤ You can also consider addressing the reasoning for strikes in general and why every work force should have the right to protest unjust working conditions by going on strike. This will necessarily take you away from the question somewhat which can be a challenge but may lead to an interesting essay. In this context it is absolutely paramount to not lose track of your argumentative chain and to relate your main body back to the question in your conclusion.

➤ You should definitely consider to use the recent junior doctor strikes as pivot point of the essay. It provides a good pivot point to organize your essay around and it will also give you real life examples of how doctor strikes can be made as safe as possible and how potential harm to patients can be reduced as much as possible.

If we truly care about the welfare of animals, we must recognise them as fellow members of our communities with their own political rights and status.

➤ This can be a quiet difficult topic to argue since the question covers a wider range of different topics that need to be addressed or at least be clear in your head in order to write a good essay.

➤ The first point to define is the idea of animal welfare. What do we understand by animal welfare and what implications does this have on the interactions between humans and animals. At this point it would be helpful to be aware of what rules exist already and what defines current considerations of animal welfare. Having a basic knowledge of this will strengthen your essay. However, if you do not have any idea of animal welfare, you can always stay on a more general and philosophical level.

➣ The second point to be clear about is the meaning of political rights and status. Make sure you have a vague idea of what this would mean and also how this could be put into action, in particular since you are required to argue that we do not need to allocate animals political right and status. Points to consider in this context are also that with right always come duties and how these can be applied to animals.

➣ In the context of this question it can also be helpful to consider the idea of conscience and intellect in animals. Try and connect this to the idea of political rights and status and the attached duties and possibilities. Taking the right to vote for example, how are cats and dogs supposed to understand what politicians say and even if they were to understand what they say, how do we know if they have the intellectual faculties to make a decision about such matters.

➣ Another avenue you might want to explore is the matter of ownership. When it comes to animals, whether they are pets or animals that themselves are a resource such as in the milk and meat industry, what role does the owner of the animal play. If we make them members of our community with political rights and status, does that make them ownerless and what implications does this have? Or do they retain their ownership and if so, how does that then impact the de facto role they take in society. Since animals will always require some degree of human support either through for example access to medical care or in order to gain access to food, how does this arrangement work form a legal perspective?

➣ In general it could be helpful for this essay title to imagine animals as humans that are somewhat limited in their ability to communicate with the rest of society and how this would shift the role they play as members of society.

➣ When it comes to political institutions again, it would be useful to have a general understanding of what institutions already exist that deal with animal welfare and animal rights and the protection and care of animals. Examples of here could be NGOs such as Greenpeace or organisations such as the RSPCA.

➣ Finally, much like the previous topic, keep in mind that this is a difficult and somewhat charged subject and that your admitting university will receive a copy of your essay that may well be discussed, at least on a theoretical level, in your interview. Thing you should avoid are extreme claims such as animal snot needing special rights since they have no mind and are just things or property etc.

END OF PAPER

2017

Section 1

Question 1: C

Start by converting everything to ml so that you don't get confused. Hugh had 900ml of yellow paint left, meaning he used (1500 – 900 =) 600ml of it. This means that he also used 600ml of red paint to create the orange paint, as they were mixed in a 1:1 ratio. If the room was 40% orange and represents (600 + 600) = 1200ml of paint, this means that the 60% pink represents 1800ml of paint. A quarter of the pink paint was red, meaning 450ml of red paint was used to make the pink.

600ml (in the orange) + 450ml (in the pink) = 1050ml of red pain used overall

1500ml – 1050ml = 450ml of red paint left

Question 2: D

A is definitely not true; there is definitely no causal evidence from this statement alone that use of antidepressants leads to *worse* outcomes for patients (i.e. we cannot know if the disability claimants are taking antidepressants or whether they represent a different population). There is also no evidence from the information that there is short term efficacy of this medication.

B is not necessarily correct; we have no idea whether doctors are being 'increasingly encouraged' to prescribe these drugs. There may be other reasons for the increase in numbers seen over time; there may be more people suffering with their mental health in the present, there may be more people seeking help for it than previously, or more people aware of the claims there are entitled to make.

C is also not necessarily correct. Similarly to above, there may be other reasons for the mental health figures getting worse over time. including an increasing incidence of mental health issues. There is a causal link between the prescriptions and claimants in this answer, which cannot be drawn from the figures alone.

D can be drawn as a conclusion from this stem alone. The figures do indeed show that on a population level, the long term mental health in the UK is declining, and that this is not improving despite increasing use of antidepressant drugs. This answer doesn't assume any causal link between the drug prescriptions and disability claimants, instead just focussing on the numbers.

Question 3: D

A satisfies the bedrooms, garage, garden, distance to grocery store; but not distance to sports facilities. 4/5

B satisfies the garden and distance to sports facilities; but not bedrooms, garage or distance to grocery store. 2/5

C satisfies the bedrooms, garage, garden and distance to sports facilities; but not distance to grocery store. 4/5

D satisfies the bedrooms, garage, garden, distance to grocery store; but not distance to sport facilities. 4/5

E satisfies the bedrooms, distance to grocery store and sports facilities; but not garage or garden. 3/5

Out of those satisfying 4/5 wishes, D is the cheapest.

Question 4: A

The key argument against nuclear power in this passage is that it 'poses and unacceptable risk to the environment and to humanity' and that stations 'create tens of thousands of tons of lethal, high-level radioactive waste.' Thus, the phrase that would weaken this argument the best would minimise these concerns.

A would weaken the argument well; it highlights that there is a way to counter-act the unacceptable risk to the environment/humanity that the author talks of.

B is incorrect; the passage suggests that we should be using less nuclear power so the author would be satisfied with this statement. It doesn't tackle the issues that are raised against nuclear power.

C gives an argument against wind power, but doesn't counter the key arguments raised against nuclear power that are highlighted above.

D is not correct; the argument actually acknowledges that nuclear power is 'less air-polluting that fossil fuels' and this is not a key reason for concern for the author.

Question 5: D

This question is obviously quite hard to explain with text alone. These questions often require trial and error and visualisation in your mind of how each shape would appear in different orientations. You are allowed to bring scissors to the exam and cut shapes out, although that may not help so much with this question compared to previous ones regarding cube folding, etc.

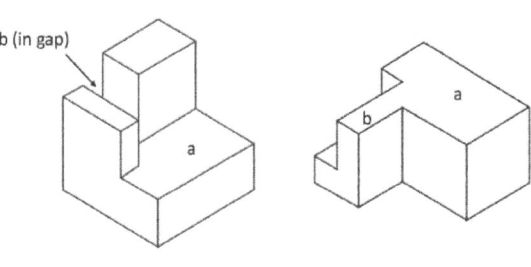

Look at the shape of 'a' on the diagram. It is nearly a rectangle with one width slightly smaller than the other. If both 'a's were appositioned directly there would be a perfect fit, whereas none of the other shapes given would be able to do this.

Also, when looking at the gap made by 'b' in the diagram, you can see it would need to be filled by a thin part of the block, which D is able to do.

Question 6: C

For any disease in medicine, there are 'risk factors' that increase your likelihood of developing a particular condition. For example, other risk factors for prostate cancer include increasing age, having a family member with the disease, or being black. However, even with no risk factors, there is a chance (albeit smaller) that one may develop the disease. Conversely, even with every risk factor for a disease, there is no guarantee that one will definitely develop the disease.

The key aspect of this argument, and simultaneously the flaw, is the suggestion that men can prevent the development of prostate cancer by minimising weight gain, as highlighted by C

A and D address other cancers which is not an issue tackled by this argument.
B doesn't address the causal link between changes to diet and exercise and prostate cancer itself.

Question 7: B

Adding up all the students at the school gets to 144, therefore there are 72 girls.
None of the girls swam and 40 girls played rounders.
28 pupils ran, of which 14 were girls.
Therefore 72 girls in total – 40 (rounders) – 14 (running) = 18 girls who played football

Question 8: C

The reconvinction frequency rate is the number of offences per 100 offenders in the cohort. Thus, over a 9 year follow-up period, there were 1057.5/100 = ~10.6 reconvictions per person in the cohort. However, the question asks specifically for the frequency of those who reoffended in the first place (74%), so we must do 10.6/0.74 = 14.3.

(Alternative method if it helps you understand it better: 42, 721 offenders in total, of which 74% were reconvicted, which is 31613 reconvicted. There were 10.6 reconvictions per offender in the total cohort, so 10.6 x 42721 = 452842 for total number of reconvinctions. If we want a figure for the number of reconvinctions per re-offender, 31613 reoffended, so we need to do 452842/31613 = 14.3)

Question 9: E
1 is true. The information explains that the figures are cumulative. 43% were reconvicted in the first year and cumulatively 55.2% by the second year, so the proportion convincted in the first year is 43/55.2 = ~0.78 = ~78%. (If you'd rather work with numbers, 43% is 18370 and 55.2% is 23582. 18370/23582 = ~78%)

2 is not true. As the figures are cumulative, 43% were reconvicted in the first year, and 61.9% by the third year, meaning only 61.9% - 43% = 18.9% were reconvicted in years 2 and 3. This is less than a third of the 74% that were reconvicted over 9 years. (Again, working with numbers, 31613 were reconvincted overall, 18370 over the first year, 26444 over three years; therefore 8074 over years 2 and 3. This is less than a third of 31613.)

3 is true. The reconviction frequency rate was 185.1 per 100 offenders at this time, meaning 1.851 per offender. There were therefore 42721 x 1.851 = 79077 reconvictions.

Question 10: C
The key information for this question is: 'offenders who received sentences of less than 12 months... committed 39% of all offences that led to a conviction in the first year of the follow-up.'

As shown above there were ~79077 reconvictions in the first year. 39% of these were by those who received sentences of less than 12 months.
79077 x 0.39 = 30840 = ~31000

Question 11: G
The wording of the question, 'might feasibly,' means that any reasonable suggestion that could account for a decline is acceptable; it doesn't need specific evidence or to be supported by the data.

1 makes sense because out of those who are going to eventually be reconvicted each year, a proportion had already done so and were in prison, so there is a smaller cohort each year.

2 is correct because we are looking at a specific cohort only (i.e. nobody can be added to the population size) and **reconvictions** rather than any new convictions. Naturally, some of the cohort will pass away.

3 could be true; if there was indeed harsher sentencing, this could feasibly deter those who would have likely reoffended with lighter sentencing.

Question 12: D

Unfortunately, there is not always a neat mathematical way to solve these types of questions; trial and error is probably best.

A cannot be true because the passage states that 'the performer who plays the role of Gracie cannot play any other characters.'

B cannot be true because both Teddy and Guard 1 are in scene 1.

C cannot be true because of the statement 'the performer who plays Rose also plays Guard 1' which would mean one performer would have to play Rose, Guard 1 and Sarah. Rose and Sarah are both in scene 10

E cannot be true because Sarah needs to be played be a female, and Graham needs to be played by a male

F cannot be true for similar reasons to C; the performer would have to play Rose, Guard 1 and Guard 2. Both guards are in scene 1.

Question 13: B

This is a classic BMAT correlation does not necessarily equal causation question. The passage even states that the drop in selenium levels *correlates* with the three extinction events.

A is nothing to do with extinction, which is the main topic of the passage.
B is correct because it acknowledges that we do not know the exact causation but that the factors could be linked.

C is incorrect because there is no mention of evidence regarding other trace elements, so we do not know how they compare in importance.
D is incorrect because it implies definite causation.

Question 14: B

The Citrons gained 57 seats and lost 29 hence now have 80 + 57 - 29 = 108. 108/240 = ~0.45
The Jonquils gained 26 seats and lost 80 hence now have 126 + 26 – 80 = 72. 72/240 = ~0.3
The Saffrons gained 51 seats and lost 25 hence now have 34 + 51 – 25 = 60. 60/240 = ~0.25
The pie chart that shows this best is B (the part which is exactly a quarter is probably most helpful).

Question 15: A

The argument presented is in the following format:
- There are two potential hypotheses for an observation, one of which is correct.
- One reason can be ruled out based on objective evidence.
- Therefore, the other reason must be correct.

A is presented in this way.
B doesn't give evidence to rule out the first potential hypotheses, only evidence to support the other reason.
C doesn't give 2 potential hypotheses for an observation.
D doesn't rule out one of the hypotheses objectively, only subjectively.

Question 16: D

All the digits add up to 38, and each digit is different. There are 8 digits in total, so each number except one from 1-9 are used. Now use trial and error to see which digit can be excluded to get to a total of 38.

A $2 + 3 + 4 + 5 + 6 + 7 + 8 + 9 = 44$

B $1 + 2 + 4 + 5 + 6 + 7 + 8 + 9 = 42$

C $1 + 2 + 3 + 4 + 6 + 7 + 8 + 9 = 40$

D $1 + 2 + 3 + 4 + 5 + 6 + 8 + 9 = 38$

E $1 + 2 + 3 + 4 + 5 + 6 + 7 + 8 = 36$

Question 17: D

The argument is very specifically suggesting that being a childhood star can cause problems in later life, so do not extrapolate this argument to include any other groups of people.

1 is not correct because the author doesn't ever argue that break-ups and mental break-downs are exclusive and unique to childhood stars; instead they are merely suggesting that the *risk* would increase as a childhood star.

2 is incorrect because the author does not suggest any link between being adored as a child and addictions/broken relationships. The author uses the word 'adored' to emotionally charge the argument rather than as a logical explanation.

Question 18: B

Cocoa powder used = 100 + 85 = 185g. 315g remaining.

Eggs used = 2. 10 remaining.

Sugar used = 330 + 200 = 530g. 70g remaining

No lemons used. 5 remaining

Milk used = 250ml. 2250ml remaining

Butter used = 400 + 150 = 550g. 50g remaining

Flour used = 400 + 225 = 625g. 375g remaining

There is only 50g of butter left, and 8 pancakes requires 50g of butter, so this is the maximum that can be made (there are no other limiting factors at this point).

Question 19: B

The claim in the headline is that a fifth of the papers contained errors in the spreadsheets. Therefore, if they are not actually errors, the support that the data gives to the claim would be weakened - this is why B is correct.

A is not correct because the headline isn't referring to any other scientific fields.
C is not correct because even if the results were , that wouldn't discount the fact that there were errors.

D is not correct because there is no way of knowing whether this would actually reduce the number of papers containing errors.

Question 20: B
1 is incorrect, we don't have data for total number of papers published for an individual year so we cannot make this conclusion.
2 is correct; looking at the graph the figure was 50 for 2009 and just above 100 for 2011
3 is not correct; Nature published 23 with errors and BMC Bioinformatics with 21.

Question 21: D
The papers with a higher % than the average (1st graph) are Nature (23 papers), Genes Dev (55), Genome Res (68), Genome Biol (63) Nature Genet (9), Nucleic Acid Res (67) and BMC Genomics (158).
Adding these together gets to 443 papers, and out of 704 this represents 63%.

Question 22: C
'The authors found that the number of genomics papers packaged with error-ridden spreadsheets increased by 20% a year over the period, far above the 10% annual growth rate in the number of genomics papers published'

Often with these proportion questions, it is easier for the human brain to convert into figures first, which doesn't actually change the calculation. So, imagine that in 2015, there were 100 papers published and 80 were affected.

2016: 80 x 1.2 = 96 papers affected. 100 x 1.1 = 110 papers published
2017: 96 x 1.2 = 115 papers affected. 110 x 1.1 = 121 papers published
2018: 115 x 1.2 = 138 papers affected. 121 x 1.1 = 133 papers published
Therefore, every paper would be affected by 2018.

Question 23: E

Looking at the shaded area, we can work out that the puzzle pieces that would fit would require 4 bits that stick out to fill the gaps and 2 that go inwards. Additionally, in the middle to join the 2 pieces, there would need to be a bit that stuck out and a part that stuck in. Therefore, in total we should expect 5 parts that stick out and 3 parts that go inwards. This is only fulfilled by E.

The diagram above, using x and y, shows one way that the pair of pieces could fit into the jigsaw puzzle.

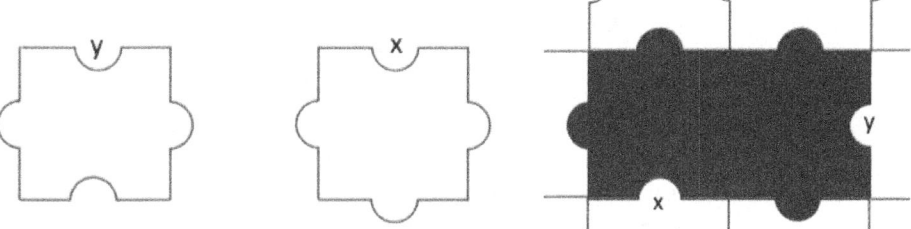

Question 24: E

The argument suggests a exclusive, causal inverse link between the number of children a woman has and their life expectancy based on a correlation. Only E acknowledges that there could be other factors that influence this correlation.

A is not correct because the argument doesn't assume or mention women's recognition of the toll of childbirth.

B is incorrect because the argument actually acknowledges that it is referring to women in rich nations.

C is incorrect because the argument is not about infant mortality.

D is not correct as the argument doesn't suggest this, only that the *risk* is increased with multiple pregnancies.

Question 25: E
The distance for the original journey between the two towns is not known, so let's call this x. We don't know the time take for the original journey, so let's call this y. Obviously, distance = speed x time.
Original journey: x = 30y
The distance is increased by 4km in the new journey, the speed is reduced by 3km/h and the journey time increases by 25%
New journey: x + 4 = 27 x 1.25y
Solve the simultaneous equations. x = 30y, and x + 4 = 33.75y so 4 = 3.75y and y = 1.067. x = 32
New journey is x + 4 = 36km

Question 26: C
The passage says that the government suggest the health checks **could** equate to prevention of over 2,000 heart attacks and strokes. However, even though the researchers identified many with risk factors, they need to follow up long-term to see whether there is actually prevention. Thus no firm conclusions can be drawn from the health checks yet, which is why C is correct.

A is not correct because we don't know if this number of heart attacks and strokes have actually been prevented.
B cannot be concluded, we don't know whether patients' health-related behaviours changed or not.
D may be subjectively true but is not specifically implied by the argument here, without the context of 'health checks'
E is incorrect, there is no suggestion to think this from the information given.

Question 27: B
The lowest common multiple of 400g, 300g and 200g is 1200g therefore Charlie would have ordered 1200g of each fish. This would make 24 plates.
3 packs of prawns are needed, and the third is free. Therefore $4.08 x 2 = $8.16
4 packs of squid are needed, and one is free. Therefore $4.08 x 3 = $12.24
6 packs of cockles, whelks and smoked salmon are needed and 2 are free for each. Therefore $4.08 x 3 x 4 = $48.96

8.16 + 12.24 + 48.96 = $69.36 in total. This is making 24 dishes, therefore 69.36/24 = $2.89 each

Question 28: E

1 is true. The second line, especially the phrase 'encourages the police officers to better regulate their own behaviour', suggests that the author thinks the 'violence' and thus level of force used can often be reduced.

2 is incorrect. The first line states that police departments across the world should use body-worn cameras, but it doesn't assume that there is any interaction between police departments in different countries.

3 is correct. The last two lines highlight this. The argument is suggesting that police-worn cameras are better because there is always a clear warning about filming from the start, which implies the assumption of those being filmed by bystanders not always being consensual.

Question 29: E

The dice, with the orientation on the left, is missing a dot from its 4, and a dot from its 6. The dice, with the orientation on the right, is missing the same dot on the 6 but we do not know which of the faces with 2 is missing a dot to make it a 3.

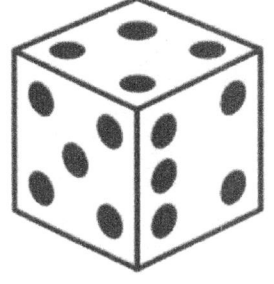 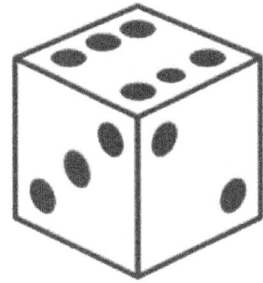

If we look at the orientation of both, the face to the left of the three dots on the 6 face must be the 5. This means the face to the left of the two dots on the 6 face must be 2 to make opposite faces add up to 7. Therefore, the dice without missing dots is as in the diagram above. Therefore, on the right dice, the bottom face is a 1, and the face that cannot be seen on the right is the 4 (with a missing dot). If you rotate this, you can get E but none of the others.

Question 30: C

This is yet another correlation does not equal causation question. Stronger brain connectivity is linked to 'positive' lifestyle traits; however, the causation may be in the other direction, or there may be confounding variables which influence both factors in the same way. Only C addresses this flaw.

Question 31: D

You can build a circle based on working out the preference of whoever is adjacent to someone. For example, on the left of Jess is someone who likes cricket and rugby, who is the same person who is on the right of David. You can go around the circle like this. Also, it helps to know that Jess is next to 2 people that share a common interest; so she must like 1 of cricket and rugby, and 1 of football and golf.

	George (F&S)	
David (C&H)		Eli (H&S)
Amir (C&R)	Jess (G&R)	Peter (F&G)

Question 32: C

This question should hopefully be straightforward, with the use of the word *'could'*. There is no evidence required but clearly both of the answers have the potential to increase the problem of London's road congestion.

Question 33: E

6 underground strikes at £10 million each = £60 million.
GVA due to congestion = £5.5 billion = £5500 million
5500/60 = 92x greater cost

Question 34: C

1 is not true. The decline of car ownership in London has occured at the same time as a reduction in London's road congestion problem, but you cannot infer a causal link.

2 is not true, there is no evidence or suggestion provided that this could be the case.

3 is true. This is heavily suggested by the third paragraph and confirmed by phrases such as 'demand for the bus service has started to decline.'

Question 35: B

To increase the GVA, there must be an increase in the production of goods and services (as per the definition).

If the widening of the congestion charge zone somehow did not increase the production of goods and services, then the proposal would not have the desired effect. With B, there may be less of the public visiting profitable retail areas (deterred by the congestion charge), meaning that the GVA may not increase – hence this is correct.

END OF SECTION

SECTION TWO

Section 2

Question 1: A
P is the gallbladder, which releases bile.
Q is the stomach, which secretes acidic HCl (thus hydrogen ions) and proteases
R is the pancreas, which secretes insulin and enzymes to digest proteins, fats and carbohydrates (protease, lipase and amylase respectively).

Question 2: E
The anode and cathode are made of copper therefore this will be the reacting species. Remember that oxidation occurs at the anode and reduction occurs at the cathode. Therefore there is the loss of electrons at the anode to generate the copper ion, and gain of electrons at the anode to convert the copper ion into the element.
(OIL RIG = Oxidation Is Loss, Reduction is Gain)

Question 3: A
1 is incorrect; microwaves have a larger (the value is **LESS** negative) wavelength than visible light. They do have a smaller **frequency**, but this is not what is stated.
2 is incorrect; all electromagnetic waves travel at the same speed through a vacuum. (This speed value is the 'c' seen in the equation $E = mc^2$).
3 is incorrect; Gamma rays have the smallest wavelength of any electromagnetic wave (it is the **MOST** negative).
4 is incorrect; X-rays are used in hospital radiography to look for broken bones.

Question 4: F
$$\left(\sqrt{5} - 2\right)\left(\sqrt{5} - 2\right) = 5 - 2\sqrt{5} - 2\sqrt{5} + 4 = 9 - 4\sqrt{5}$$

Question 5: G

This question is about the conversion of DNA into proteins, which requires both transcription and translation.

Humans have 2 alleles of every gene, one from the mother and one from the father. These can be the same, or different, and can be either recessive or dominant. The particular allele represents the exact DNA code; that is the order of each nucleic acid base (A, C, G, T) in the DNA. This is converted to mRNA by transcription, and then each triplet of bases in the mRNA code is read and converted into a specific chain of amino acids. The exact amino acid encoded, influenced by the order of bases, can influence things like the tertiary structure of the final protein and thus the shape of the active site of the enzyme.

In this disease, any of these steps could go wrong (and thus be different to normal) to give a faulty enzyme which is unable to produce healthy white blood cells, therefore all the answers are correct.

Question 6: D

1 contains 16 protons (atomic number), therefore 18 neutrons (to give a mass of 34) and 18 electrons (to give a 2- charge).
2 contains 17 protons, therefore 20 neutrons and 18 electrons.
3 contains 18 protons, therefore 22 neutrons and 18 electrons.
4 contains 19 electrons, therefore 20 neutrons and 18 electrons.
5 contains 20 electrons, therefore 20 neutrons and 20 electrons.

Question 7: F

1 is correct. The rate of evaporation increases with the temperature of the liquid because molecules have more kinetic energy and move faster on average, thus more can escape.

2 is incorrect. Still air would cause the air above the puddle to become saturated. Windier conditions allow more evaporation because there is the maintenance of a gradient between high water concentration and low water concentration above the puddle.

3 is correct. The increased surface area means that more molecules can escape at the same time.

Question 8: A
We want to pick a patient suffering for a migraine twice, so we use AND and times together the 2 probabilities.

The probability of picking the first patient is 5/20; if this occurred the probability of picking the second would be 4/19.
Therefore 5/20 x 4/19 = 20/180 = 1/9

Question 9: E
There is water in all the experiments and glucose in 2, 3 and 4. Even with no/minimal gradient, random entropy means that both water and glucose will move through the partially permeable membrane, and there will be some (~equal and opposite) movement in the other direction to equilibrate.

Question 10: C

This is a classic metal + acid à salt + hydrogen reaction

$Mg + 2HCl$ à $MgCl_2 + H_2$
As the reaction occurs, the magnesium chloride and hydrogen are formed (the latter causing the bubbling) which reduces the concentration of the reactants.
Therefore, only 2 is correct. The activation energy is irrelevant (this regards the start of the reaction) and the particles do not have less energy, it is just a concentration issue.

Question 11: C
Remember, in series, the current is always the same at each resistor (hence 4 is true), whereas the total voltage and the total resistance is additive. 2 is correct because using $V = IR$, doubling the resistance at R_1 with an equal current means that the voltage must be doubled here.
(In parallel, the voltage is constant and the current is additive.)

Question 12: F
Firstly, you can rule out A/B/C as PS is clearly over 1.8cm!
Thanks to QT and RS being parallel, the traingles PQT and PRS are proportional to one another. That means the ratio of PT:QT is the same as PS:RS. Let's call PT x and the proportion between the sides y.

x = 0.3y and 1.8 + x = 1.5y therefore 1.8 + 0.3y = 1.5y and 1.8 = 1.2y. Thus y is 1.5 and x is 0.45.
PT is 0.45cm therefore PS is 2.25cm.

Question 13: E
1 is true. The diploid cell contained 54 chromosomes therefore the haploid gamete cell must have contained half, which is 27.

2 is true; early embryonic cells need to be able to produce every different cell type in the body from an un-differentiated state, and they are therefore regarded as stem cells. 3 is not true. The gametes that are used at the start must have been produced by meosis to become haploid (and then become diploid again upon fusion).

Question 14: E

1 Fe (0) + $CuCl_2$ (+2; -1 -1) à $FeCl_2$ (+2; -1, -1) + Cu (0)

2 Cu_2O (+1 +1; -2) à Cu (0) + CuO (+2; -2_

3 Cl_2 (0) + H_2O (+1, +1; -2) à HCl (+1; -1) + HClO (+1; +1; -2)

4 $BaCl_2$ (+2; -1, -1) + Na_2SO_4 (+1, +1; +6; -2, -2, -2, -2) à $BaSO_4$ (+2; +6; -2, -2, -2, -2) + 2NaCl (+1; -1)

5 Hg_2Cl_2 (+1, +1; -1, -1) à Hg (0) + $HgCl_2$ (+2; -1, -1)

As you can see, there is reduction and oxidation of Cu in 2, Cl in 3 and Hg in 5

Question 15: F

Nuclear fission comes up quite regularly in BMAT questions and you just need to re-member how it works.

When an atom of U-238 is exposed to neutron radiation, its nucleus occasionally cap-tures a neutron, making it U-239. It then needs to undergo two β decays which con-verts 2 neutrons into 2 protons, now giving the atomic number for plutonium.

Question 16: A

Just be careful with using standard form, and simplify your calculations as much as possible (e.g. 3.6/7 à 3.5/7 to make 0.5) and you should be fine. Firstly you can re-arrange to get M = gR^2/G.

$R^2 = 6 \times 10^6 = 36 \times 10^{12} = 3.6 \times 10^{13}$

$gR^2 = 10 \times 3.6 \times 10^{13} = 3.6 \times 10^{14}$

$gR^2/G = 3.6 \times 10^{14} / 7 \times 10^{11} = \sim 0.5 \times 10^{25} \sim 5 \times 10^{24}$

Question 17: G

This question refers to coronary arteries on the surface of the heart.

1 is not true; glucose cannot freely diffuse from the blood stream, it requires *facilitated* diffusion with specific transporters.

2 is true, arteries carry blood away from the heart at high pressure.

3 is true, there are smooth muscle cells in the tunica media of the arterial vessels to allow vasodilation and vasoconstriction.

Question 18: C

You can count each element on both sides of the equation to see if it is balanced, which works for A-C, whereas D and E have other problems.

A: 7C 12H 5O 1Mg à 6C 12H 5O 1Mg

B: 4C 6H 5O 1Mg à 4C 7H 5O 1Mg

C: 7C 12H 7O 1Mg [?] 7C 12H 7O 1Mg

D: The formula for propanoic acid is not correct

E: Hopefully intuitively you can see that $Mg_3C_3O_2$ is not a compound likely to form; it would require a C_3O_2 ion to be 6-...

Question 19: E
It takes 0.01s longer for the sound wave to travel to the far wall than the near wall. The microphone is placed next to the sound source, so the sound must travel to the wall and back before it is detected.

Distance to be reflected from near wall: 2 x 2 = 4m

Distance to be reflected from far wall: 8 x 8 = 16m

Therefore it takes 0.01s to travel an extra 12m. 12/0.01 = 1200m/s

Question 20: E
Make the denominators the same so that you can add and subtract. Times the top and bottom of the first by x-1, the second by 2x, and the third by 2(x-1)

$$\frac{1}{2x} + \frac{1}{x-1} - \frac{1}{x} = \frac{x-1}{2x(x-1)} + \frac{2x}{2x(x-1)} - \frac{2(x-1)}{2x(x-1)} = \frac{x-1+2x-2x+2}{2x(x-1)} = \frac{x+1}{2x(x-1)}$$

Question 21: D
Males and females are affected similarly, ruling out this being an X-linked inheritance pattern.

A female and male with freckles are able to produce offspring without freckles, showing that it cannot be inherited recessively. Thus it is inherited in an Autosomal Dominant fashion.

Take F to be the allele for freckles and f the allele for no freckles.

Parent 1 is Ff and 2 is ff, so the offspring have a 50% chance of being either Ff (freckles) or ff (no freckles).

Parent 5 is Ff and 6 is Ff, so the offspring have a 25% chance of being FF (freckles), 50% chance of Ff (freckles) or 25% chance of ff (no freckles).

Question 22: B

Mr of hydrated copper(II) sulphate is $64 + 32 + (16 \times 4) + 10 + (16 \times 5) = 250$
Mass/Mr = $10/250 = 0.04$ moles of hydrated copper sulphate in $100cm^3$
Therefore, in 1 dm^3 (which is $1000cm^3$), there would be 0.4moles. Conc is 0.400 mol/dm^3.

Question 23: F

Newton's third law states that forces come in pairs, if object 1 exerts a force on object 2, then object 2 exerts an equal and opposite force on object 1. So if the floor is exerting force P on the table, there must be an equal and opposite force which would be the force that the table exerts on the floor.

Question 24: C

Length of the third side of the triangle using Pythagoras's theorem is
$$\sqrt{(9^2 - 6^2)} = \sqrt{45} = 3\sqrt{5}$$
Area of the triangle is $\frac{1}{2} \times 6 \times 3\sqrt{5} = 9\sqrt{5}$
Area of the circle is $\frac{1}{4}\pi 6^2 = 9\pi$
Therefore, together $9\pi + 9\sqrt{5}$

Question 25: G

1 is not correct. The gene is inactive at warmer temperatures, but this is not the same as it denaturing. (Remember denaturing is generally irreversible so if this gene denatured, it would never be active again and the cat could never get darker).
2 is correct. In the colder environment, the enzyme is active which causes the coat colour to darken, which is why the extremities of the body are darker.
3 is correct. The gene confers the potential to have a darker coat, and whether the gene is active or not depends on the environment.

Question 26: B

$2Na + H_2O$ à $Na_2O + H_2$
Mass/Mr = $0.23/23 = 0.1$moles of sodium, hence 0.05 mol H_2
Volume = n $\times$ 24 = $0.05 \times 24 = 0.12dm^3$

Question 27: C

For a straight line graph, y = mx where m is the gradient. y is the kinetic energy and x is the square of the speed which we can sub in below.

$KE = 0.5mv^2$. We have the mass to sub in as 2.5kg, so $KE = 1.25v^2$ and $y = 1.25x$, so the gradient is 1.25.

END OF SECTION

SECTION THREE

Section 3

'He who has never learned to obey cannot be a good commander'. (Aristotle)

➤ This quote is referring to the quality of leadership. Some may believe that good leaders were 'born to lead' and have always had the relevant characteristics and strengths to become an effective, charismatic leader. However, Aristotle argues that the best of leaders are those who have learnt to lead by developing their attributes and assets based around other successful leaders.

➤ As with any profession or role in life, natural talent is not enough for success. A talented sports player will need to follow the advice and potentially strict rules of their coach if they are to thrive and potentially become a professional. A 'gifted' musician or writer will still need to work hard and learn from other successful pioneers in their profession in order to prosper. Leadership is an art form like any other and without learning from others talented in this art it would be difficult to succeed.

➤ Moreover, if one has not experienced something for themselves, they are less likely to be able to be good at it. For example, it is hard for someone who has never rode a bike to teach someone else, or someone who has not had kids to give advice about mothering. In a similar vein, until one has experienced good leadership themselves and has understood what it feels like to be led well, it would be difficult to truly know whether one's own leadership is good or not. Also, it is important to understand what it feels like from the 'other side'; that is, the empathy allowed by previously being commanded should help leadership.

➤ One could argue that there are other factors that are more important in a leader than learning how to follow, and that these can be developed independently. For example, you could elaborate on some of these points:
   o Ability to inspire confidence and provide direction
   o Planning, organising and setting targets
   o Listening, supporting and giving constructive criticism if relevant
   o Accepting responsibility for mistakes
   o Being assertive and always looking forward
   o Managing time, risk and people well

➤ You could link this quote back to medicine in the conclusion; and although they can't mark you down for an opinion, possibly err on the side of arguing that learning to follow is key to be a good leader. As a doctor, one starts with foundation training where every decision is reviewed and checked by a senior doctor, and where it is vital to follow the experience of someone who as worked for many years more. This 'leader' should hopefully also teach many attributes of the job that cannot be taught from a book at medical school. In order to thrive as a doctor, and then become a good leader in the future as a consultant, one must take on board all the advice that is given to them early on in the job.

The only moral obligation a scientist has is to reveal the truth.

➤ At its most basic level, science can be considered as the pursuit of truth. The scientific method involves systematic observation, experimentation and the formulation, testing and modification of hypotheses; all scientists should use this empirical technique if they are to be successful at their role. This statement suggests that using scientific research in order to advocate for a particular way of thinking, or other roles such as educating the public, are not a moral obligations of a scientist.

➤ It is clear cut that the role of a doctor is to look after their patients, the role of a lawyer is to represent their client in legal matters; similarly, the role of a scientist is considered to be using experimentation to acquire knowledge. One could argue that the role of scientist is solely to reveal the truth, as this is what their expertise is, and then the role of others with varying professions, such as policy makers and politicians, to decide how that truth is applied and used. Moreover, some may believe that advocacy may hurt the credibility of scientists; by having a preconception of how things should be, they may consciously or unconsciously bias their experimentation in a particular way (although strictly speaking, using strong scientific methods should minimise thus, such as the use of double blinding and randomisation in a clinical trial).

➤ There are events in history whereby successful scientists have used their power and privileged position to go beyond their pursuit of truth and harm others. A few examples:

    o   Dr Reiter and Dr Wegener (both who have diseases named after them) were German physicians who committed war crimes under the Nazi regime by authorising medical experimentation on concentration camp prisoners

- o The USSR communist party set up secret laboratories where scientists could work freely against ethical restrictions; for example, an experiment whereby the head of a puppy was stitched onto the lower body of an older dog.

➢ One could argue that a scientist has the moral obligation to advocate for a particular scientific truth, especially when there could be a major danger to society. An example could be the case of global warming. Despite much rigorous scientific data showing that increasing carbon dioxide levels in the are causing atmospheric temperature increases, many politicians and global influencers deny the changes. As such, many countries and governments are not taking steps to reduce their emissions, which will make things worse and may eventually cause destruction of the planet as we know it. If scientists publically came out to promote and support changing our lifestyles to save the Earth it may significantly improve things for the generations below; that is, the potential of making the world a better place means taking action an ethical obligation.

➢ Also, one could argue that a scientist has a moral obligation to educate others and/or lead. They have likely developed a thorough, deep understanding in their area of expertise and it would benefit society for them to spread this knowledge. Alternatively, one could argue that if their research is publically funded, i.e. paid for by the public, they have an obligation to give back to the public via education.

➢ You could conclude by arguing that the baseline moral obligation of a scientist is to reveal the truth and to be a good scientist (especially if this is their sole job description), but that the best and most influential people are those who are able to successful apply (or at least think of how to apply) their knowledge, and those who are willing to educate the public.

The health care profession is wrong to treat ageing as if it were a disease.

➣   The statement is arguing that because ageing is a natural, normal and inevitable process which everyone must go through, whereas disease is an abnormal deviation from the norm which only affects a proportion of the population, we should not equate ageing as a disease. That is, something that is universal cannot be abnormal.

➣   Instead of considering ageing as a disease, it may be more useful for the health care profession to consider ageing as a risk factor for chronic diseases, and then target the specific pathology caused by that disease (which is associated but not solely caused by the ageing).

➣   Another reason to not consider ageing as a disease may be due to its certainty. Some may believe that treating ageing as a disease would lead to the misallocation of limited resources to a futile cause, which may just prolong periods of pain and/or illness.

➣   In contrast: disease is defined as a disorder in structure or function of a bodily system causing harm, and with this definition, ageing does seem to fit the bill (if a healthy adult human is considered 'normal'). For example, ageing is associated with:

      o   Bones become more brittle, muscle mass decreases, joints degenerate and become less flexible
      o   Wrinkling of the skin, greying of hair
      o   Hearing loss, loss of near vision
      o   Cognitive decline, potentially leading to dementia
      o   Cardiovascular changes, increase risk of cancer
      o   Inability to control bowel and bladder movements

➣   Moreover, if we treat ageing as a disease that can be treated and prevented, we can use scientific research to target fundamental pathways in this process, and potentially find methods to halt or slow its development. That is, treating it as a disease legitimises medical efforts to try and cure it or eliminate other conditions associated with it. Before the advent of vaccinations and antibiotics, it was rare to live over forty years old; by targeting ageing itself there is the potential to make us even more healthy.

➣   Targeting fundamental ageing mechanisms rather than 'age-related disease' may be beneficial to medicine; it may be futile to fight chronic diseases without striving to first understand their ultimate cause. Like with other diseases, modern experimental techniques have found molecular targets and deleterious changes related to ageing: particular genes involved in the process, and structures at the ends of chromosomes called telomeres which act as biological clocks for human cellular ageing. People's bodies age at different rates according to an interaction between genes and the environment.

➤ The goal of biomedical research is to enable people to be as healthy as possible, for as long as possible. With modern technology and methodology, it should be possible to better delineate the exact pathways involved in ageing. If we found more good evidence that ageing is a preventable or curable process, then it would make a lot of sense to treat it as such and fund and develop procedures to slow the process. However, in contrast, if the evidence suggested that resources were better spent directly targeting specific pathologies in age-related conditions, then it would not be worthwhile to treat ageing as a disease.

END OF PAPER

Afterword

Remember that the route to a high score is your approach and practice. Don't fall into the trap that *"you can't prepare for the BMAT"*– this couldn't be further from the truth. With knowledge of the test, time-saving techniques and plenty of practice you can dramatically boost your score.

Work hard, never give up and do yourself justice.

Good luck!

Acknowledgements

Thanks must go *Somil* for his tremendous help in putting these set of answers together and to *David* for lending his expertise with the trickiest of questions.

Rohan

About UniAdmissions

UniAdmissions is an educational consultancy that specialises in supporting **applications to Medical School and to Oxbridge**.

Every year, we work with hundreds of applicants and schools across the UK. From free resources to our *Ultimate Guide Books* and from intensive courses to bespoke individual tuition – with a team of **300 Expert Tutors** and a proven track record, it's easy to see why UniAdmissions is the **UK's number one admissions company**.

To find out more about our support like intensive **courses** and **tuition**, check out **www.uniadmissions.co.uk/bmat**

SECTION THREE

Your Free Book

Thanks for purchasing this Ultimate Guide Book. Readers like you have the power to make or break a book –hopefully you found this one useful and informative. *UniAdmissions* would love to hear about your experiences with this book. As thanks for your time we'll send you another ebook from our Ultimate Guide series absolutely <u>FREE</u>!

How to Redeem Your Free Ebook

1) Either scan the QR code or find the book you have on your Amazon purchase history or your email receipt to help find the book on Amazon.

2) On the product page at the Customer Reviews area, click 'Write a customer review'. Write your review and post it! Copy the review page or take a screen shot of the review you have left.

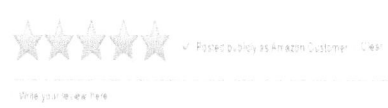

3) Head over to www.uniadmissions.co.uk/free-book and select your chosen free ebook! You can choose from:

✓ The Ultimate UKCAT Guide
✓ The Ultimate BMAT Guide
✓ The Ultimate Oxbridge Interview Guide
✓ The Ultimate Medical School Interview Guide
✓ The Ultimate Medical Personal Statement Guide
✓ The Ultimate Medical School Application Guide
✓ BMAT Past Paper Solutions Volume 2
✓ BMAT Practice Papers

Your ebook will then be emailed to you – it's as simple as that!
Alternatively, you can buy all the above titles at

www.uniadmissions.co.uk/our-books

BMAT Online Course

If you're looking to improve your BMAT score in a short space of time, our **BMAT Online Course** is perfect for you. The **BMAT Online Course** offers all the content of a traditional course in a single easy-to-use online package – **available instantly** after checkout. The online videos are just like the classroom course, ready to watch and re-watch at home or on-the-go and all with our expert Oxbridge tuition and advice.

You'll get full access to all of our BMAT resources, including:

✓ 8 Full Practice Papers, Worked Solutions
✓ Copy of our acclaimed book "The Ultimate BMAT Guide"
✓ Full access to extensive BMAT online resources including:
✓ 800 practice questions
✓ Fully worked solutions for all BMAT past papers since 2003
✓ 10 hours of BMAT on-demand lecture series
✓ Ongoing Tutor Support until Test date – never be alone again.

The course is normally £99 but you can get **£ 20** off by using the code "*UAONLINE20*" at checkout.

https://www.uniadmissions.co.uk/product/bmat-online-course/

£20 VOUCHER:
UAONLINE20

UKCAT Online Course

If you're looking to improve your UKCAT score in a short space of time, our **UKCAT Online Course** is perfect for you. The **UKCAT Online Course** offers all the content of a traditional course in a single easy-to-use online package – **available instantly** after checkout. The online videos are just like the classroom course, ready to watch and re-watch at home or on-the-go and all with our expert Oxbridge tuition and advice.

You'll get full access to all of our UKCAT resources, including:

✓ Copy of our acclaimed book "The Ultimate UKCAT Guide"
✓ Full access to extensive UKCAT online resources including:
✓ 6 Full Practice Papers, Worked Solutions
✓ 1250 practice questions
✓ 10 hours of UKCAT on-demand lecture series
✓ Ongoing Tutor Support until Test date – never be alone again.

The online course is normally £99 but you can get **£ 20 off** by using the code *"UAONLINE20"* at checkout.

https://www.uniadmissions.co.uk/product/ukcat-online-course/

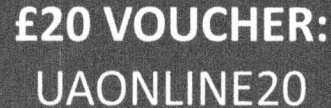

£20 VOUCHER:
UAONLINE20

Medical Interview Online Course

If you've got an upcoming interview for medical school but unable to attend our intensive interview course– this is the perfect **Medical Interview Online Course** for you. The Online Course has:

✓ 40 medical interview on-demand videos covering Oxbridge and MMI-style questions.

✓ Copy of the book "The Ultimate Medical Interview Guide."

✓ Over 150 past interview questions and answers.

✓ Ongoing Tutor Support until your interview – never be alone again

The online course is normally £99 but you can get £20 off by using the code "*UAONLINE20*" at checkout.

https://www.uniadmissions.co.uk/product/online-medical-interview-course/

£20 VOUCHER: UAONLINE20